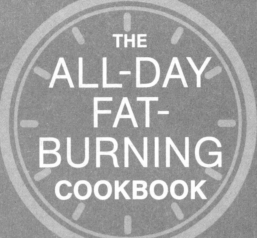

THE
ALL-DAY
FAT-
BURNING
COOKBOOK

TURBOCHARGE YOUR METABOLISM WITH MORE THAN
125 FAST AND DELICIOUS FAT-BURNING MEALS

THE
ALL-DAY
FAT-
BURNING
COOKBOOK

YURI ELKAIM

RODALE

RODALE
wellness

Live happy. Be healthy. Get inspired.

Sign up today to get exclusive access to our authors, exclusive bonuses, and the most authoritative, useful, and cutting-edge information on health, wellness, fitness, and living your life to the fullest.

Visit us online at RodaleWellness.com
Join us at RodaleWellness.com/Join

© 2016 by Yuri Elkaim and Elkaim Group International, Inc.
Photographs © 2016 by Rodale Inc.

Rodale books may be purchased for business or promotional use or for special sales. For information, please write to:
Special Markets Department, Rodale Inc., 733 Third Avenue, New York, NY 10017

Printed in the United States of America
Rodale Inc. makes every effort to use acid-free ♾, recycled paper ♻.

Photographs by Mitch Mandel/Rodale Images
Clock illustration by Shutterstock
Book design by Amy King
Food styling by Carrie Ann Purcell
Prop styling by Stephanie Hanes

Library of Congress Cataloging-in-Publication Data is on file with the publisher.
ISBN 978–1–62336–607–0   hardcover
Distributed to the trade by Macmillan
2   4   6   8   10   9   7   5   3   1   hardcover

🌱 RODALE.

We inspire health, healing, happiness, and love in the world.
Starting with you.

Dedicated to my wife, Amy, and our three boys,
Oscar, Luca, and Arlo,
who are always my best food critics.

And a special thanks to the thousands of women and men
all around the world who've been enjoying my simple
and delicious fat-burning meals for years.

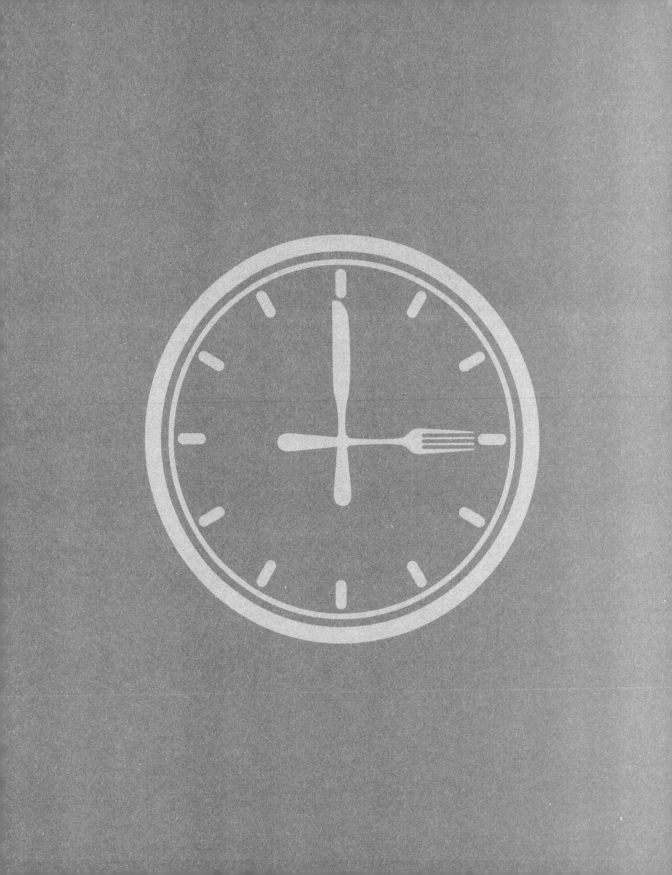

Contents

Introduction

MY BIO READS LIKE A FAIRY TALE.

I'm a registered holistic nutritionist, fitness and fat-loss expert, and the *New York Times* best-selling author of *The All-Day Energy Diet* and the precursor to this book, *The All-Day Fat-Burning Diet*. In my early twenties, I was able to pursue my childhood dream of playing professional soccer. Later, I acted as the strength and conditioning and nutrition coach for men's soccer at the University of Toronto for 7 years.

I've appeared almost everywhere in the media, including on *The Dr. Oz Show* and *The Doctors* and in *Huffington Post* and *Men's Fitness*, and I've been fortunate to have helped more than half a million men and women transform their bodies and health over the past two decades. But don't be fooled by the glossy bios and write-ups that make me seem more than human. The reality is that I'm just a husband and father who's struggled for years with my own cravings and bad food habits.

It all started when I was a young boy growing up on man-made processed foods, take-out, fast-food restaurants, and 2-minute microwave dinners. I rarely ate vegetables or fruit and instead navigated my way toward copious amounts of bread, cereal, pasta, and cheese. Not many colors were in my diet. It was pretty white and very unhealthy.

As the years went by I suffered with terrible asthma, eczema, and really low energy. I remember eating Shreddies cereal topped with 2 tablespoons of sugar and 2% milk only to find myself experiencing terrible stomachaches for hours afterward. As a teenager, I had no idea what I was doing and I wasn't clued in to how these symptoms would eventually change the course of my life forever.

I won't bore you with the entire story, especially since I've described it in detail in my previous books, but here's what happened in a nutshell: At the age of 17, I lost all of the hair on my body in just 6 weeks to an autoimmune condition called alopecia. At the time, neither I nor my doctors had any idea why this happened, but the answer surfaced after several years. As with almost all health problems, including carrying too much body fat, I discovered that what you eat is a major factor. Duh! It took me until my midtwenties to figure this out, and only after going back to school to study holistic nutrition.

Since then, I've overcome most of my health issues and regrown my hair and lost it again several times, as tends to be the way with autoimmune conditions. But more importantly, I've been able to empower a lot of people to take better control of their health and finally lose weight without overhauling their lives with my simple and realistic approach to eating and living well. Yet, even after all this, I've still battled with my own dietary demons lurking in the closet from my unhealthy childhood eating habits. Pizza, burgers, fries, and chocolate are just a few of my vices and, on occasion, I'll give in and enjoy them.

Even though I've never struggled with being too heavy, I've helped thousands of men and women who have. I understand the struggles that you've faced. Perhaps you've eaten well and exercised regularly, yet still that stubborn fat wouldn't budge. Or maybe, like me, you've been held hostage to food cravings for most of your life, especially when things get really stressful. And I get it if you feel like you're "out of control" with your diet, like someone else inside of you is running the show. Whatever your struggle, I'm going to do my very best to help you put an end to it with this cookbook. Yes, that sounds like a bold claim, and perhaps we won't completely eliminate what's been holding you back from losing weight and keeping it off, but we will certainly come close.

I Love Food. Do You?

Okay, so it's confession time for me.

Unlike many other "perfectly healthy" gurus out there who seem to never slip with their diets, I'm no dietary saint. Yes, I eat well most of the time and love foods that make me look and feel my best, but I've also cut myself a little more slack over the years. During the past 10 years, I've tried pretty much every diet out there so I could better relate to my overweight clients who were considering the very same diets. Unfortunately, like so many others, I ended them within a few days or weeks simply because they weren't realistic and sustainable—at least not for me.

I'm a self-proclaimed "healthy foodie." I love great food. Even though I encourage eating gluten-free and more plant-based foods, you won't find me at a nice restaurant turning away a delicious steak tartare spread over nicely toasted crostini with a touch of Dijon mustard and a pickle on top. Mmmm.

When people ask me if I'm paleo or vegan, I remind them that I don't believe in labels because they really limit us in this world. I consider myself a "healthatarian" (I guess that's a label, isn't it?) who simply eats real food in a way that resonates with my body, while occasionally (I mean weekly) allowing myself to go off course. I want to encourage you to do the same—if that works for you. And in this cookbook, I'll show you how to do that without further ruining your metabolism.

For us (you and me), it's all about progress, not perfection. It's about the process, not just the outcome. It's about enjoying what we're eating, no matter what that may be, because the guilt and negative energy we project into our food could well be worse than the food itself. I really want to make sure you know what this journey is all about, because it's not about being hard-core anything. It's about embracing every imperfect step you take toward a healthier and happier you. Missed a green smoothie today? No worries! Skipped the salad and went straight for pizza? Don't worry about it. Pick yourself up and start fresh tomorrow. Is tiramisu your favorite dessert? It's certainly mine!

Sure, I'm not recommending you eat these foods (at least the latter two) on a regular basis if you want to look and feel your best, but I believe that these "bumps" along the way make it a beautiful journey. We don't sit in our car in the parking lot scarfing down that burger. We don't hide in our closet to scarf down the occasional piece of cake. We enjoy food around a table with our family and friends. There is no food shaming or guilt. Just enjoy the damn food! It's all about being a better version of ourselves every single day. I think my "Be My Best" manifesto says it best.

How I do anything is how I do everything.
So "I can't" doesn't exist in my world.
I am fit, healthy, and happy because I do.
Perfection isn't my goal. It's giving it everything I've got.
That's good enough for me.
And if that means failing, that means learning.
Because I'll always be growing and daring to be my best.

This is my life, so I refuse to be a passenger in it.
I strive to make tomorrow better than today.
I savor my successes.
I learn from my mistakes.
I embrace new challenges.
And whatever life brings, I make it count.
Because I'll never give up on being the best version of myself.

We are all meant to shine.
So I do what I can to lead by example.
I exercise because I enjoy it, not to repent my dietary sins.
I seek balance in what I eat, not confining dogmatic diets.
I find happiness in moments of mindfulness.
I let myself be vulnerable.
And I love who I am.
Because the ultimate success in life is being my best self
and knowing that that's good enough.

Do This at Home to Live Longer

Did you know that research shows that elderly people who cook most of their meals at home live longer than those who do not prepare the majority of their food at home?[1] Cooking your own food gives you much greater control over what goes in it. You can make healthy ingredient swaps if you care to; you can also control portion sizes and the freshness of the ingredients when you're cooking for yourself.

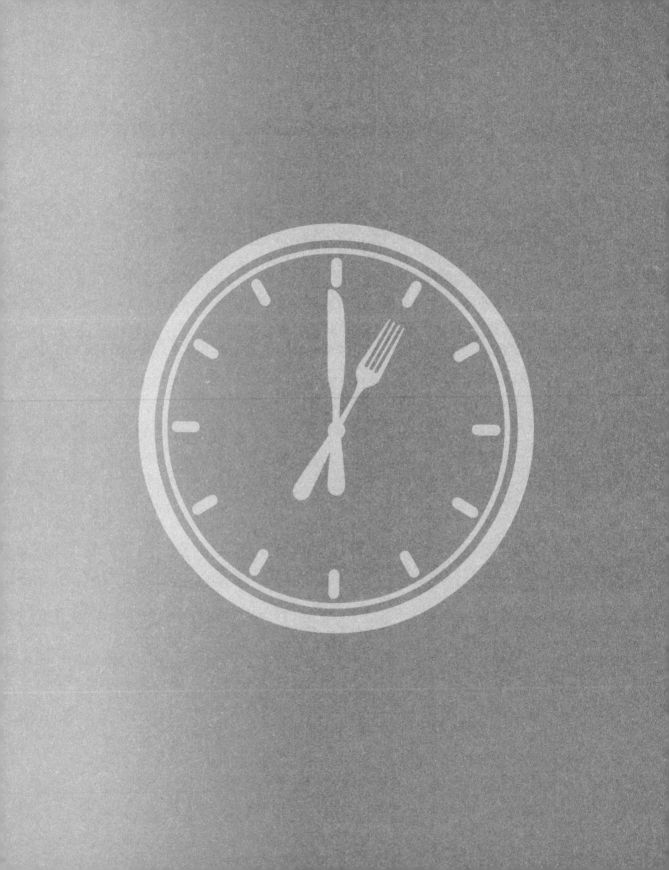

Chapter 1

All-Day Fat-Burning Principles

MAYBE YOU'RE READING THIS BOOK because you've followed my work for some time. Perhaps you've seen my videos on YouTube, or maybe you just loved *The All-Day Fat-Burning Diet* and are eager for more amazing recipes that jibe with our proven 5-Day Food-Cycling Formula. Whatever the case, welcome! Throughout this cookbook I'll share a number of success stories from readers of *The All-Day Fat-Burning Diet* (the predecessor to this cookbook) who have seen incredible health and weight-loss breakthroughs following these principles. I know they'll inspire you. And before you jump ahead to the quick, fat-burning, gourmet-style recipes in this cookbook, I think it's important to lay the foundation of what makes this program so effective at helping you lose weight. That's what we'll cover over the next few pages.

Readers, Start Your Engines!

Welcome to the recipe-centered sequel to *The All-Day Fat-Burning Diet*. I know you're going to love the recipes I've got in store for you in this cookbook. But before we jump in, I think it makes sense to bring you up to speed on what all-day fat-burning is all about, especially if you didn't read *The All-Day Fat-Burning Diet*. Once you know the philosophy behind what we're doing here, you'll be able to eat this way for life.

After all, this is not a *diet*; it's a way of living. Once you understand it and try it, you'll see how easily it can become part of your daily fabric. There are very few rules, no calories or points to worry about, and there's no deprivation. With this approach, you get to eat like a champ and look and feel like one too. In this chapter, we'll recap why we're fat, revisit how the All-Day Fat-Burning 5-Day Food-Cycling Formula works, and explain how to use this cookbook so you get the

---

Kayla's Transformation

"I am not a good dieter at all! I have always been 'skinny fat' and have been able to eat pretty much whatever I wanted. The past few years I have put on 10 to 15 pounds each year and kept them on. After hearing Yuri's podcast with Lewis Howes, I decided to buy Yuri's *The All-Day Fat-Burning Diet*.

"Despite being 'skinny fat,' I was always unhappy with my body, even from an early age, and I wanted to change that. My original goal was to lose 10 pounds in 21 days, but when I lost 7 in the first week, I decided I needed a new goal! My first 21 days ended on Super Bowl Sunday 2016 and, after a weekend of eating unhealthy food, I could not wait to get back to my healthy and delicious meals!

"Going into my second 21-day cycle, I am aiming to lose 20 more pounds. After reading *The All-Day Fat-Burning Diet*, I felt fully equipped to change my eating habits for life. Thank you, Yuri Elkaim! I am on my way to finally being happy with my body, which is the ultimate prize!"

most out of it. I'll also answer some common questions about this program and its recipes.

Recap: Why We're Fat and the Secret to Burning Fat 24/7

As I discussed in detail in *The All-Day Fat-Burning Diet*, the major reason we're fatter than ever before is because our body feels threatened by life's numerous stressors, including the foods we eat, the way we exercise, our lack of quality sleep, and our mental and emotional state. When our body feels that its survival is at risk, it slows down its metabolism to conserve energy and store fat. It's a hardwired, built-in mechanism that comes with being human. This trait helped us survive 100,000 years ago, but in today's world of excess food and endless stress, our primitive makeup doesn't stand a chance.

To make this a little more scientifically clear for you, most of the foods at our disposal nowadays (think everything outside of fresh foods like vegetables, fruits, legumes, nuts, and healthy animal products) create a cascade of inflammation inside our body. As a way of protecting itself, our body's adrenal glands pump out cortisol to cool the inflammation. However, since cortisol is a major stress hormone, its constant presence tells our brain that our body is out of balance and that its survival could be at stake (it isn't really, but that's what our body believes). As a result, our metabolism slows to a halt, fat burning stops, and the body buckles down as if getting ready to hibernate for the winter.

Please understand that it's not just food that creates this stress response. Anything that knocks your body out of homeostasis (its state of balance) on a consistent basis will lead to the same result. Negative emotions, lack of sleep, too much exercise, the wrong foods, environmental toxins, and unhealthy gut bacteria are just a few of the culprits that stress our body. And all of this, over time, wreaks havoc on your metabolism and puts most of your hormones out of whack. That's why it's so tough to lose weight and keep it off.

I want you to remember that unless you've been eating fast food every single

Sit Less and Stand More

One of the fat triggers I discussed in *The All-Day Fat-Burning Diet* was *sedentarism*: too much sitting. Here's one more reason to get off your butt and spend more time standing and moving around: A 2009 study of 17,013 men and women between 18 and 90 years of age revealed that daily time spent sitting was associated with an elevated risk of all-cause and cardiovascular disease mortality! Basically, the more you sit, the higher your risk of disease and early death. And these results were independent of any extra physical activity levels and body mass index. The results of this study remind us that losing weight and staying healthy don't just revolve around going to the gym a few times per week but rather reducing the amount of time we spend sitting.[1] If you're deskbound, then set a timer to go off every 20 minutes to remind you to stand up, take a little walk (or move around), and do some light stretches. Or try alternating 30 minutes of standing with 30 minutes of sitting while at work. It will pay off big-time in the end.

day and have no intention of moving your body on a regular basis, your inability to lose weight is not your fault.

You've picked up this cookbook not for my charming good looks or my quirky Canadian humor, but because you're committed to living healthy. You want a body you can feel proud of. Perhaps you want to be able to walk into your favorite clothing store, try on anything you like, and love what you see in the mirror. Perhaps you want to feel sexier and more confident in your own skin. Or maybe you want to avoid going down the same diseased road as some of your family or friends who've battled with their weight for far too long.

Whatever your reason for losing weight, I believe that you've done your best to eat relatively well and exercise regularly up until this point. Maybe you've slipped along the way, but it's okay—we all have. So if the weight still hasn't budged, then I'm sure you can appreciate that burning fat is a little more involved than eating less and exercising more. It requires eating clean foods and cycling them in a way that resonates with and honors your body's natural rhythms. I firmly believe (and have observed) that if we can work *with* our body instead of *against* it, we'll have a much easier time losing weight and feeling our best.

We are part of nature. And just as everything in nature has a natural flow to it, so does our body. The waves crashing on the beach, the changing of the seasons, the warming and cooling of the earth—everything in life has an ebb and flow. We shouldn't consider ourselves separate from this. Our body is governed by circadian rhythms; failing to honor them will be as catastrophic as a surfer who mistimes catching a 30-foot wave. For instance, cortisol *should* be highest in the morning and lowest at night. Melatonin, our sleep hormone, *should* be lowest in the morning and highest at night. Growth hormone *should* be secreted in highest quantities during deep sleep, and on and on.

When we eat and live in a way that disrupts these natural patterns, our health and waistline suffer. Fat loss is an internal process largely determined by the health of your hormones and your body's natural rhythms. If you don't support these inner workings, then no amount of calorie cutting, counting, or insane exercise will make any lasting difference. Does that make sense?

Count Your Blessings

We live in the most amazing time in history, with more freedom, choices, and luxuries than ever before. Yet most people are still miserable, which works against their chances of making favorable choices that will improve their health. The good news is that taking just a few minutes each day to count your blessings and express gratitude for what's working well in your life goes a long way to improve your happiness, self-esteem, and long-term well-being, according to research in the journal *Applied Psychology: Health and Well-Being*.[2] And when you feel better, you make better decisions that support your ultimate goals. Try writing one page in a journal each night about things you're grateful for, including your health, your family and friends, the roof over your head, the ability to read this book, and whatever else comes to mind. There's so much to be thankful for, and when you truly *feel* that, stress melts away and happiness increases.

The beauty of *The All-Day Fat-Burning Cookbook* (and the original diet behind it) is that it provides a realistic, proven, and sustainable framework for eating healthy and delicious foods that lower inflammation and stress in your body and honor your body's natural rhythms without making you feel deprived or requiring you to spend all of your time in the kitchen. What you'll find in this cookbook are fat-burning meals so fast and delicious you'll think they're bad for you. And they'll all be organized for you in alignment with the 5-Day Food-Cycling Formula that I laid out in the predecessor to this cookbook. Following these recipes, within this proven food-cycling framework, will turbo-charge your metabolism, blast away pounds, and help you enjoy food once again. And remember, there's no counting calories, weighing your food, or any other unsustainable dietary rituals. Just enjoy the recipes on the right days and you'll be fine.

Revisiting the 5-Day Food-Cycling Formula

In *The All-Day Fat-Burning Diet,* I laid out a proven 5-day formula for cycling your calories and carbs to help reset your body's metabolism to lose up to 5 pounds per week. As a reminder, the reason for developing this method is that humans were most likely hardwired to do best with fluctuating periods of feast and famine. And so it's a way of eating that resonates more closely with our inherent metabolic makeup.

Our Paleolithic ancestors did not have the luxury of refrigerators, 24-hour

Start Your Day with Lemon Water

Squeeze the juice of a lemon half into 500 milliliters of water (about 2 cups) and make that your first drink of the day upon waking. Lemon has an alkalizing effect on your body, which helps to awaken your digestive system and flush out toxins that have built up overnight. You'll also find that it helps you pass your first bowel movement of the day more easily, which is great for keeping your gut clean and happy.

convenience stores, fast food, or coffee shops on every corner. They lived and thrived in a slightly more unpredictable environment where they might experience abundance on some days and scarcity on other days (or times of the year). Yet today, we've been brainwashed to think that we need to be eating every few hours or else our metabolism will shut down. That's simply nonsense, and I talk about the dangers of following this advice in *The All-Day Fat-Burning Diet.*

Here, I want to quickly remind you of how my proprietary 5-Day Food-Cycling Formula works, since you'll see the recipes in this book organized according to this system. The best part is that it's a very natural and intuitive way of eating for which your body will thank you.

The 5 days are as follows:

1. Low-Carb Day
2. 1-Day Feast
3. 1-Day Fast
4. Regular-Cal Day
5. Low-Cal Day

To follow the plan, simply follow the above sequence for 5 days, and then repeat. Once you've done this cycle once or twice, it will feel intuitive and natural. Plus, it will help you tap into what your body really needs so that, over time, you can truly understand when you can eat more and when you can—and should—eat less based on your body's hunger signals.

We know that one of the only ways to extend life span and lose weight permanently is through frugal eating—essentially, to eat less. But no one likes doing that. Eating less in many cases means depriving yourself and feeling hungry. For most of us, that's not a sustainable way of living. This 5-Day Food-Cycling Formula allows you to tap into the health benefits of frugal eating without actually feeling like you're eating frugally. Sure, there's a day of fasting every 5 days, which we won't concern ourselves with in this cookbook, but otherwise you'll be eating delicious foods that provide your body with a ton of nutrients, while helping to reset your body's out-of-whack hunger hormones so that you're not constantly needing to eat.

I'd like you to keep this 5-day plan in mind as you go through your days—not in a fanatical way but rather as a reminder to be a little more conscious of your food choices. The good news is that simply following the recipes in this cookbook will keep you on track. Here's a quick review of how the 5-Day Food-Cycling Formula works.

DAY 1: LOW-CARB DAY

GOAL = less than 50 grams of net carbs on this day

- Avoid starchy carbs and fruit.
- Eat protein at each meal.
- Make fats your main energy source on this day.
- Eat unlimited amounts of fibrous veggies.
- Eat when you're hungry, and stop when you're 80 percent full.

Net carbs are simply total carbs in a food minus the fiber. So, if a food has 50 grams of total carbohydrates and 20 grams of that is fiber, then the net carbs would be 30 grams. Make sense? I'm not expecting you to count this stuff when preparing your meals. All of the low-carb meals in this cookbook have already taken this all into consideration. Plus, if you just follow the first guideline above—avoid starchy carbs and fruit—on this one day, then you'll easily stay under your 50 grams of net carbs on your Low-Carb Days. Don't make it more complicated than that.

The reason we limit carbs for this one day is to allow your body to tap into your fat stores, instead of glycogen (stored carbs), for its fuel. Doing so also helps your body become a better fat burner instead of a sugar burner that is constantly craving sugar and carbs. However, it's important to also understand that going low carb for even just a few days can have negative consequences on your thyroid and thus your metabolism. That's why we use only one Low-Carb Day every 5 days with this approach. It's much safer and just as effective.

DAY 2: 1-DAY FEAST

GOAL = a minimum of 250 grams of net carbohydrates and up to 50 percent more caloric intake than on your Regular-Cal Days

- Eat healthy feast foods ad libitum—without feeling guilty.
- Don't binge or stuff yourself; eat until you're 80 percent full, not to the point of discomfort.
- Eat your biggest meal after you work out.
- If you can't eat more at any given meal, then graze throughout the day on nuts, fruit, or other healthy foods.

This day serves to revive your metabolism (especially your thyroid and the hunger hormone leptin) after your Low-Carb Day and to prepare it for the upcoming 1-Day Fast. This isn't a "cheat day" but rather a day that is focused on eating more healthy carbohydrates (since they are important for many hormonal functions) and increasing your overall food intake. You don't want to stuff yourself or feel uncomfortable. Simply find ways to add a little more food into your day by snacking between meals, using slightly larger portion sizes, and/or eating richer, more calorically dense meals. Again, no need to worry about the details—just eat more than you normally would, so long as you're hungry and not keeling over in a food coma.

To give you a basis for comparison, 1 cup of beans provides about 125 grams of carbohydrates, which is half of your requirement for this day. One banana provides about 30 grams of carbs. So you can see how quickly (and easily) this would add up. Throughout the cookbook, you'll see certain recipes that are marked "Feast Approved," which indicates that they are naturally higher in good calories, carbs, and healthy fats. This is not to say that you can't have any other recipes on your 1-Day Feast but just that these specific ones will provide "more feast per forkful."

DAY 3: 1-DAY FAST

GOAL = nothing but water and herbal teas for 18 to 24 hours

- Consume nothing but water or herbal tea. It's that simple.
- If you're taking any supplements (multivitamins, fish oil, etc.), give your body a break for this one day.
- Probiotics and digestive enzymes are okay to take, since they can provide systemic benefits in the absence of food.

This day doesn't really concern us in terms of the recipes in this book. It's pretty self-explanatory—don't consume any food for 1 day. I detail many health and fat-loss benefits from doing this in *The All-Day Fat-Burning Diet*. However, here, let me just give you a quick rundown of the best way to do a 1-Day Fast.

To make it easy on yourself, simply start your fast after dinner on your 1-Day Feast so that by the time you wake up the next morning you've already completed about 12 hours of your fast. Then, if you can make it on water and/or herbal tea until midafternoon or early evening, you're golden.

Having coached thousands of people through this process, let me say that being hard on yourself for not making it the full 24 hours is not a good idea. Don't beat yourself up. If you've fasted 14, 17, 20, or however many hours, just be happy with the fact that you've given your body a "breather" to do some much-needed cleansing and healing. Please remember that your first 1-Day Fast will likely be a challenge, especially if you're used to eating all the time. However, it will also be one of the most rewarding experiences you go through as you learn a lot about why you eat.

Much of the time, you'll recognize that you're not hungry but rather anxious, bored, or in a "conditioned" situation (like working at your desk) where you would normally be snacking on food. This awareness alone is worth doing a 1-Day Fast. For more guidance on how to incorporate this fast into your week, simply follow Chapter 13, The 10-Day Metabolic Reset, which includes two fasts over the 10-day period.

DAY 4: REGULAR-CAL DAY

GOAL = to establish a baseline

- Eat as you normally would.
- Eat when hungry, stop when 80 percent full.

Hillary Succeeds in Spite of Skepticism

"When I signed up for the first All-Day Fat-Burning Diet beta test group in December of 2014, my goal was to get into my favorite *very* tight skinny jeans that I couldn't even button anymore. I thought there was *no* way this would happen in just 21 days. So although I was excited to get started, I was just a bit skeptical. It was the holidays after all, and the temptation to eat junk food was all around me. I followed the plan pretty much to the letter (with a few exceptions at some holiday parties), and by Day 21, not only could I zip up my favorite jeans, but there was about half an inch to spare! I was floored! I only weighed myself two times and decided to let my clothes do the talking.

"I noticed that I felt satiated all of the time and stopped craving chips, sugar, coffee, and alcohol. As a fantastic added bonus, my energy levels soared, my borderline blood sugar issues disappeared, and I just felt lighter and happier! I have stuck with the plan off and on for 14 months and every time I go off the cycle I notice all of my old symptoms come creeping back. I have been following the plan for about 6 weeks now and feel absolutely amazing! Thanks, Yuri, for giving me hope and confidence to make this a lifestyle. It is truly a gift!"

This day is as close to your current "normal" day of eating as you can get. We're not counting calories or measuring stuff, so try to instinctively get a feel for how much you normally eat. This becomes your baseline for your Regular-Cal Day. It doesn't have to be perfect—close enough is good enough. From this baseline, you can better determine how much more to eat on your 1-Day Feast and how much less to eat on your Low-Cal Days.

DAY 5: LOW-CAL DAY

GOAL = to eat fewer calories than your baseline

- Aim to eat about 25 percent less than you did the day before (your Regular-Cal Day).
- Eat more raw foods, light soups, and smoothies.

The Low-Cal Day is pretty straightforward, although many people report that this is the toughest day to wrap their heads around. Since the goal is to consume about 25 percent fewer calories than on your Regular-Cal Day, you want to focus on foods that are nutrient rich but low in calories. That's why salads, light soups, and smoothies can work really well here.

How to Use This Cookbook

This cookbook is not just an array of recipes. It's strategically arranged to build upon *The All-Day Fat-Burning Diet* so that you have an ample number of delicious fat-burning recipes that take less than 20 minutes to prepare for each of the days within the 5-Day Food-Cycling Formula that you are not fasting.

You can use this cookbook two different ways.

1. Follow the recipes in accordance with the 5-day plan so that you enjoy recipes for each of the various days on those specific days. For example, on your Low-Carb Days you would use recipes in this cookbook designated "Low Carb." On your feast days you would enjoy pretty much any of the recipes (especially those higher in starchy carbs), and so forth. Since I want to make your life a little bit easier, I've also included the

10-Day Metabolic Reset for you (see Chapter 13). This is a meal plan that lays out a very specific eating schedule over 10 days (incorporating the 5-Day Food-Cycling Formula) to get you back on track, while reducing the need for you to think about what to have for dinner or any of your other meals.

2. Enjoy any of the recipes whenever you like. This is generally how most cookbooks work. Sift through the pages, find the recipes that look appealing to you, and make those whenever you like. This is less strategic but still totally fine, since all of these recipes will support your health and help you trim your waistline.

In addition to awesomely delicious recipes, you'll enjoy some cool features throughout, such as simple tips and tricks to make you more proficient in the kitchen, eye-opening facts you never knew about many of the foods you'll be eating in these recipes, and simple, small actions that can turn into lasting habits for a healthier, happier, and leaner you.

Common Questions

Here are some of the most common questions I've been asked since *The All-Day Fat-Burning Diet* hit store shelves. Since most apply here as well, I thought the answers would be of value to you.

Why are The All-Day Fat-Burning Diet *recipes so helpful for losing weight?*

Losing weight is not as simple as eating less and moving more. What's holding back people who follow that rule and still can't lose weight is an internal physiology gone wild. The human body inherently knows how to stay lean, but only when our internal workings are ideal. Thus, the goal is to reset our body's innate "factory settings" so that it can do its job properly. The recipes in this cookbook help to make that possible. Here are two big reasons this program works so well.

1. Eating differing amounts of food each day is a more natural state of eating for most people and acts to reestablish ideal hormone function.

2. Eating clean foods reduces most of the fat triggers at the root of weight gain, most notably inflammation.

What if I'm paleo or vegan? Can I still follow these recipes?

Great! This book is diet agnostic. About half the recipes in this cookbook contain animal products, but whether you're vegan, paleo, or anywhere in between, you can easily follow the food-cycling guidelines and food principles to suit your needs.

I'm vegan and wondering what I can eat on Low-Carb Days. What do you recommend?

That's a good question, because almost all high-protein vegan foods—think legumes—are also relatively high in carbohydrates. Thus, low-carbohydrate days are a bit tricky for a vegan. I'd recommend eating plenty of fibrous vegetables and increasing your intake of healthy fats to compensate for the lower number of low-carb vegetarian protein options. Nuts can also be enjoyed to increase your protein and fullness on a Low-Carb Day.

Can I follow these recipes if I have diabetes, high blood pressure, or another health concern?

Yes, following these recipes will not only help you lose weight but, as a by-product, will improve your overall health. Plus, all the recipes are well balanced, have a low-to-medium glycemic load, and contain no artificial junk. The recipe ingredients are just real food and the dishes, quickly made from scratch, will improve your health. Of course, always consult your doctor before beginning this or any eating plan.

Will the recipes take forever to make?

No, the recipes in this book take 20 minutes or less to prepare. Some require additional cooking time, but your hands-on work will always be less than 20 minutes.

Which foods am I not allowed to eat?

I'm not your boss, so I can only recommend that you eat and avoid certain foods. For best results, and to truly follow the program, I recommend you avoid dairy (organic,

Save Your Adrenals by Ditching the Caffeine

Thousands of readers of *The All-Day Fat-Burning Diet* asked me if coffee was okay to drink on the plan. My answer, no matter what diet you're following, is usually no. The reason for that is because caffeine is a stimulant that activates your adrenal glands to pump out more stress hormones like cortisol and adrenaline. Over time, combined with the extra stressors from daily life, your adrenals can eventually wear out, leaving you looking and feeling exhausted. When this happens, losing weight and keeping it off becomes very difficult. Instead, swap the coffee for a decaf (Swiss water processed) or an herbal tea. I'm a big fan of holy basil tea, which is known to help revive tired adrenals and bring a sense of calm to your body—much better than feeling that artificial caffeine high, if you ask me.

grass-fed butter is the exception), gluten, and soy. Clean animal products, vegetables, fruits, nuts, beans, and legumes are perfectly fine.

Do you recommend consuming coffee or caffeine?

I would strongly advise against caffeine, since regular consumption of this stimulant, combined with an already stressed-out life, will deplete your adrenals and wreak havoc on your blood sugar levels, leaving you feeling exhausted and requiring even more caffeine to function. At the minimum, switch to a decaf coffee or use herbal teas.

Will I have to give up any of my favorite foods?

If your favorite foods are ice cream, pizza, hot dogs, and French fries, then probably you will. Otherwise, *The All-Day Fat-Burning Cookbook* is gluten- and dairy-free, low in sugar, yet still loaded with delicious meals that take little to no time to make.

How many meals should I be eating per day?

We now know that it doesn't matter how many meals you eat each day. As long as total calories remain roughly equal, there is zero impact on your metabolism or your ability to lose weight if you have as little as two or as many as five meals. So, if you've been led to believe that you need to eat every 2 to 3 hours to keep your metabolism humming, then that's simply false. If you've got diabetes or blood sugar problems, ask the advice of your health care professional, but eating more frequently is probably recommended. However, assuming you're adequately healthy, you should only eat when you're hungry and stop when you're 80 percent full. If you follow that simple rule, then you'll know exactly how often to eat throughout the day in a way that works for you.

Why Are You Here?

Many people asked why I decided to write a cookbook. For one, creating simple and delicious fat-burning recipes has been one of my claims to fame for years. And I'm excited to share an arsenal of brand-new fat-burning meals with you in this book! The other reason for writing this cookbook is that I wanted to provide a good variety of quick, mouthwatering meals that make you feel like a hero in the kitchen. I realize you may not have all day to spend in the kitchen, but that doesn't mean you can't enjoy gourmet-quality meals in a matter of minutes. You're probably busy and you're most likely not a professional chef. Yet you still want great-tasting food that does your body good, right?

Good news: I'm not a chef either. I'm just a regular guy with a background in nutrition who discovered through trial and error how to make healthy food taste amazing. And now I'm here to share that knowledge with you. Plus, I try to spend as little time as possible in the kitchen—ironic, since I love great food. I've got three little boys and a busy life, so I don't have all day to spend preparing food. I'm sure you can relate. You're probably busy too. Maybe you've got kids and are driving them around from one commitment to the next. Perhaps you're tired of feeling deprived and relying on fad diets that make you eat rabbit food or meals that taste like cardboard. You might be a lot like me and just want delicious meals that help you look and feel your best without fussing about counting calories, weighing your food, or having to spend a lot of time. And perhaps, like many of my clients, you just want to curb cravings and find a way to make healthy eating tasty and a consistent part of your life so you can once again have a healthy relationship with food.

Whatever your goal, one fact remains: What you put on the end of your fork matters. And if you read the predecessor to this cookbook, *The All-Day Fat-Burning Diet*, then you know that you *can* eat delicious food that is really good for your waistline and your health without counting calories or feeling deprived. And that's exactly what you'll get in this cookbook, doable recipes for the novice and expert chef alike. You don't need to be a pro to make these meals, although your taste buds will think you are once they taste your amazing creations.

Why This Cookbook Is Different

I want to be very clear with you: This cookbook is *not* like most other cookbooks you might already have. First and foremost, one thing you will not find in this cookbook is the calorie or nutritional breakdown for any of the recipes. I don't believe in counting calories and fussing about how many grams of healthy fat are in a food. Yes, full-fat coconut milk is loaded with fat—but it's extremely good for you. Our bodies are so messed up metabolically partly because we've been obsessed with reducing fat (even healthy fat) in our diet. Doing so robs our body of the necessary building blocks for healthy hormone production, among other things.

Here, you'll find a focus on the whole food, where we enjoy food in its entirety—not fractionalized components. I believe this is a much healthier way of viewing our food. Plus, when you focus on quality, the quantity of your food matters less. And if you're still worried about calories, grams of carbs, and portion sizes, then keep in mind that all of that has been taken into account for you. For instance, your low-carb meals all have low net carb counts, which makes those recipes suitable for your Low-Carb Days. They've also been labeled as such. In fact, where applicable, you'll see labels like "Low Carb," "Low Cal," or "Feast Approved." These give you a quick indication that a specific recipe is suitable or recommended for that specific day in the 5-day cycle. You can enjoy recipes that don't have such labels on any day.

Finally, I need to remind you that *you've* got to put in the work. Even though

Macy Is Back in Control of Her Diet and More Confident Than Ever

"I am the healthiest 17-year-old I know, and yet somehow I'm also one of the bigger ones. Everyone around me can eat whatever, whenever, and wherever and not work out. I would exercise two times a day and eat super healthy, and still not lose weight. Before *The All-Day Fat-Burning Diet,* I was already eating 'healthy.' This means no sweets or soda and very limited processed foods. And yet somehow I was gaining weight. I had tried every plan there is to make you lose weight. It would work for a few weeks, then I would gain it (and more) back! Not okay!

"I was sick and tired of being so self-conscious about what others thought of my body. I found out a few weeks before I started this program that I have hypothyroidism. So I knew I had to watch what I ate carefully because of my slow metabolism. Another roadblock in my journey. This program became more than just a way to lose weight for good. It was also a confidence-builder.

"After 21 days, I lost 1 inch off my hips and butt, 1½ inches off my stom- ach, and ½ inch around my thunder thighs! In just 21 days! That got me so excited, it called for a happy dance full of a confidence I didn't have before! It may not seem like a lot, but I don't have much to lose compared to oth- ers. I am in my own battle. I'm 5'3" and 130 pounds, most of it being in my butt and thighs. They stick out in everything I own, making it impossible to buy new clothes.

"Every day in this program is another way for me to fight for what I want. It's a way for me to be in control of what I eat and to not feel badly about eating when I am hungry for fear of gaining weight. I don't step on the scale two or three times a day anymore, and somehow I know I have lost weight and am keeping it off, even though I'm eating more than ever before and exercising far less. And *losing weight!* This has truly been a life-changing way to live. Not just a phase. It's a lifestyle I enjoy. I may never 'beat' my hypothyroidism, but now I know how to live and manage it, while getting the body and confi- dence I want. Thank you, Yuri!"

I've done my best to make these meals simple and quick to make, *you* are the one who has to take a few minutes each day to prepare them. I've done everything for you except shop, chop, and cook your food. But you have to be willing to make it. Knowing how to prepare great food is one of the most basic and valuable skills any human can develop. If making toast is the extent of your kitchen know-how, then your kitchen confidence will soar once you make these meals. You'll never want to go back to your old ways. I hope this clears the air and gives you a better idea of what to expect as you sift through these pages.

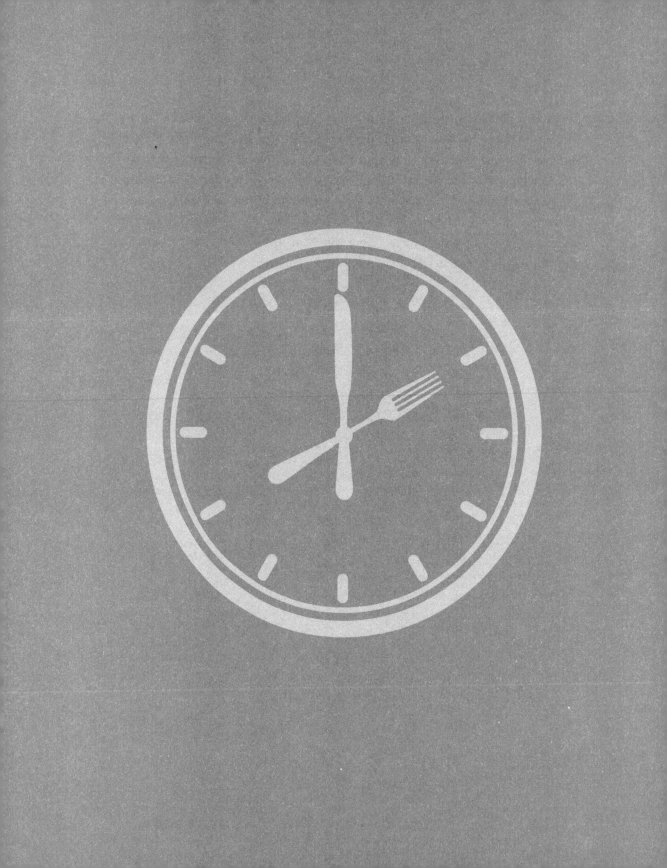

Chapter 2

How to Make Healthy Eating Stick for Life

I DON'T JUST WANT TO GIVE YOU A COOKBOOK full of great recipes that you might use occasionally. I want to equip you with the tools to make eating this way doable for life. After all, I've observed that most people feel frustrated when they aren't consistent with their healthy eating endeavors, which negatively affects their confidence and optimism about trying new things that could lead to big breakthroughs in their health. I've included this chapter to keep you from falling into this common dietary sinkhole. And if you already have, then consider this the ladder to help you get out.

You're Not Alone

If you're like most of my clients, it's not eating healthy that's difficult; it's eating healthy consistently that's the real challenge! If you find yourself constantly starting over or saying "I'll start again tomorrow" every time you try to eat healthy, then what I'm about to share with you is going to change that for good.

In this chapter, I want to give you some tangible strategies that will help you incorporate the All-Day Fat-Burning Diet recipes (or any other healthy recipes) into your life and make them stick. After all, there's no point in doing something for just a few days, right? I want you to enjoy lasting results, and that comes down to creating the right environment and habits to help you do that. That's what I'm going to show you how to do here. But before we jump in, I want to clear up a few myths you may have heard about eating healthy.

Myth #1:
A healthy diet has to be boring and bland

As I've already mentioned, I'm a self-proclaimed "healthy foodie." I refuse to give up delicious food, so every recipe I create is at least as enjoyable to eat as the unhealthy alternative. In this cookbook, you won't feel deprived or like you're dieting. Not only will you love my recipes, they'll energize you, help you burn more fat, and make you look and feel amazing.

Myth #2:
A healthy diet takes longer to prepare

This is a *huge* myth that is simply not true. In fact, all of the amazing recipes I'm going to share with you take 20 minutes or LESS to prepare. You probably can't even make it to your local McDonald's and back that fast. With three young boys, a wife, and a business to run, I don't have a lot of time to spend in the kitchen, and I'm sure you don't either. And even if you have the time or enjoy spending your days in the kitchen, I'll show you some cool ways to become more proficient so you can impress yourself and others with your culinary skills.

Myth #3:

To have a healthy body, you must be fanatical about your diet and block specific foods out of your life forever

This is something a lot of nutritionists and other diet "experts" preach. Yes, *The All-Day Fat-Burning Diet* and this cookbook are about removing allergenic foods that cause inflammation—foods like gluten, dairy, and soy, for example. But that doesn't mean you need to feel deprived. There are countless alternatives that are tastier and healthier than the common foods we're so often drawn to. My goal is not to tell you that you can never have those foods ever again, but instead to help you experience how good you can look and feel when you choose alternative foods.

Once you feel the difference, you won't want to go back to those foods of old. Just one piece of bread and you'll probably feel like taking a nap. A glass of milk and you'll likely feel bloated. Is it really worth it? This is not about giving things up but about *choosing* to enjoy better foods. You're worth it. In fact, I have a confession to make. I'm not 100 percent gluten- or dairy-free. I definitely recommend doing your best to eliminate these foods, but if you slip up occasionally, don't beat yourself up. You're only human.

In my house, Amy (my wife) and I have developed an extremely effective system that makes healthy eating easier while minimizing cravings without condemning certain types of foods. A large part of that system is having amazing recipes like the ones in this book, along with an environment that supports clean eating behaviors (more on that in a moment). Plus, we don't want our kids growing up in a Nazi-style home where they're condemned for wanting or eating a specific food. In the long run, I believe that does more harm than good, as they develop negative food associations that are no healthier than the supposedly unhealthy foods they occasionally might eat.

When you follow a system you can rely on—like the one in this book—you create a predictable outcome, which will make reaching your health goals much easier and far less stressful. You don't have to give anything up forever. You've got to live your life. Just do your best to make choices that make you look and feel your best.

One of the reasons most people "fail" when embarking upon any kind of diet is that they often feel deprived. When you think you'll never have something again, you have to rely on willpower, which only lasts so long before you crack and end up back at square one.

My goal for you is to have a system in place with delicious recipes that are "brush your teeth" simple to make so that relying on fleeting willpower is not your strategy for eating healthy consistently. The goal is to make this endeavor a healthy habit that becomes so automatic that you rarely have to think about it. And I'll help you do that with the strategies in this chapter. Let's start by looking at three important steps you need to take.

Step 1: Set Up Your Environment to Win

Setting up your environment to win is massively important in helping you get the results you're after. If your kitchen looks like a war zone, then you'll have a hard time finding the clarity of mind to think straight, let alone cook. Therefore, it's important to keep your kitchen clean and tidy.

Clean it up. There's something about having a clean environment that eases your mind and reduces stress. Another reason a clean kitchen is important is because environment always trumps willpower. For example, if you have a cake sitting on your countertop, left over from a party, what will you do? Throw it out? Most of us wouldn't because we're so invested in the monetary value of that cake, or any other food. We hang on to it. However, if your goal is to eat healthy so you can stay slim and lean, is this setting up your environment to win? I think you know the answer is an absolute no. Unless chocolate cake improves your health (which, unfortunately, it does not), you need to remove it and any other negative influences. This is a big part of setting up your environment to win. The whole idea is to make unhealthy choices very inaccessible.

Consider the following three scenarios.

Scenario 1: You have a chocolate cake sitting on the counter. Ease of access is a no-brainer. You can just go by, grab a knife, cut yourself a slice, and it's ready to eat. When you get home after a long day and you're stressed out and just want that carb fix, the chocolate cake is right there, tempting you.

Scenario 2: You don't have the cake at home, but you can go to the store, which is a couple blocks away, and buy it. The unconscious thought process goes something like this: "Ugh, I have to get my shoes on and walk or drive over. Then, if I drive, I have to park the car, then get out of the car and go into the store. I have to buy the cake, then get back in the car and drive back home. Then I have to take it out, cut a slice, and then I can finally eat it." As you can tell, going through this process is more work, so it's less likely you'll eat the cake in this scenario.

Scenario 3: You don't have to go to the store, but you have cake mix in your pantry. Now if you want the cake, you have to preheat the oven, take out the cake mix, find a large bowl, get the eggs, the milk, mix it all together, take out the pan, pour it into the pan, then throw it into the oven for 30 minutes.

Thirty minutes later, the cake comes out of the oven. Then you have to let it cool before you put the icing on top. Then, an hour after the start of this entire process, you're ready to eat. Just like with Scenario 2, that's quite a journey and a lot more work than simply plowing into a cake that is sitting on your counter, ready to go. So do you see where I'm going with this? No matter which foods you want to remove from your diet because you know they're holding you back, the key is to make unhealthy food options far less accessible. When you do, you'll be less likely to eat them. We're naturally lazy creatures, so this is one of those instances where you want to embrace your natural human laziness and make it work for you. Get rid of the junk. Go through your fridge and pantry and chuck the cookies, ice cream, breads, and other foods that don't jibe with our All-Day Fat-Burning guidelines. Remember, this is not about deprivation but about making a conscious choice to no longer settle for a less-than-optimal diet that leaves you looking and feeling like crap.

I'm sorry to say this, but hoarders are not the picture of health. That's because how you do anything is how you do everything. If your kitchen is a mess, then so are you. Sorry, but it's the truth. Getting the results you want (in any area of your life) is all about standards. If your kitchen is a disaster, then please recognize that that's where your transformation begins. When you give yourself more respect and refuse to settle for anything less than awesome, then naturally you will want to be surrounded by a more inspiring environment that reflects who you truly are.

If you have trouble giving yourself a little more self-love, then just start by cleaning up your kitchen. Put away the dishes, organize your cupboards, get all the unnecessary stuff off the counter. When you're done, you'll feel so much better. Seriously. And that's because we're happiest when we make progress. If you turn your war-zone kitchen into a clean and tidy haven, you will have made incredible progress and you'll feel great about that. You'll never want to go back to your old ways. And along with that will come better food choices to support your new, higher standards that you've set for yourself. Make sense?

Aside from cleaning up properly, there's one strategy that will keep your kitchen tidy and your life more peaceful.

Create organizational systems. You need systems so that when you go to the grocery store and come back with a couple bags of groceries, you know where everything goes; this way, your kitchen doesn't look like a disaster zone due to the huge onslaught of groceries. If you go to the store and buy almonds, beans, spinach, or apples, each of these foods should have a designated place in your kitchen. You should already know where to put them so you don't have to figure it out every time you get home with groceries. Put the vegetables in one drawer, meat in another, and so on. There are no set rules for where you *should* put things, so create an organizational system that works for you. Same deal for silverware, cutlery, plates, and cups. Pick where those things should go and stick to it. Keep those areas clean, organized, and free of crumbs or other mess.

This isn't about being obsessive or a neat freak. You just want your kitchen to be clean and organized in a way that's conducive to healthy eating, so eating well becomes effortless. When you live in a space that is clear of clutter, you feel better, and when you feel better, you make better decisions. Between cleaning up your kitchen and getting rid of the junk that could be holding you back, you've

Three Simple Tips to Make Healthy Eating a Little Easier

Tip #1: Make desired behaviors easier

For example, if you want to juice more, leave the blender out and ready to go instead of tucked away. Cut up veggies ahead of time so you can tear into them when you're hungry. Keep them ready to go in the fridge, so when you get home after a long day and your willpower is down and you don't feel like thinking about what to make for dinner, you can turn to the cut-up veggies instead of giving in to the bag of chips. If you feel like you need a bit of salt, drizzle a little sea salt on the veggies, and that'll quench that craving. Small adjustments like this that cut down the number of steps in healthy habits will dramatically increase your chances of sticking to them.

Tip #2: Make bad influences very inaccessible

We talked about this in the cake example: It's extremely important to make the bad influences as difficult to access as possible. If your weakness is eating toast, don't buy bread and put away the toaster, so it's a pain to get it out and set it up.

Tip #3: Have satiating foods like healthy fats and protein powders readily available

If you suffer from cravings, this is one powerful tip. It will save you over and over again when you get those blood sugar drops throughout the day and want that quick sugar fix. If you have some healthy fats ready to go, like coconut oil or olive oil, you can simply eat a tablespoon and you'll feel more satiated and relaxed, avoiding the need for the deadly carb fix. This will also give your body lasting fuel to energize you and help you power through the rest of the day.

I also recommend having protein powder on hand. Protein has the highest thermic effect of all the macronutrients and keeps you full longer than fats or carbs. Protein powder is my "secret sauce" for preventing and combating late-night and afternoon cravings. Plus it only takes about 10 seconds to make a delicious protein shake, which increases your metabolic rate to help you churn through more calories. Plan for those moments of weakness by always having a simple protein powder on hand as your secret weapon. If it tastes really good (without added sugars), then that's even better.

now created a winning environment. This is very important because, as I mentioned earlier, your environment will always trump willpower.

You can have the most determination possible and commit to not eating junk, but when you get home at the end of a long day and your willpower is at its lowest, that's when you are likely to give in to temptation. You need your environment to support you when you're at your worst, because here's the thing about willpower: It's much like the battery on your smartphone. It dwindles down the more you use it. The more decisions you make throughout the day and the more temptations you resist, the more willpower you use, which eventually drains your body's ability to resist temptation. I'll show you some scientific proof for this notion in a few pages when we talk about creating healthy habits that stick.

But you know what I'm talking about, right? You get home at the end of a long, tiring day and you just want dinner done. You certainly don't feel like lifting a finger to make it. It's okay; I've been there too. And if you're living in a messy environment, that only adds more fuel to the fire. You get that feeling that says, "Ah, screw it, I'm just going to order pizza." It's all too easy to give in to carbs, chocolate, or chips because you don't have a plan in place (i.e., knowing exactly what you're having for dinner) and your environment is not set up to support you at your weakest. Willpower can only take us so far, so please do your best to follow my advice and make your kitchen fat-burning friendly. In conjunction with the recipes and meal plan in this cookbook, you'll be armed with a bulletproof strategy to no longer rely on willpower and finally be on your way to food freedom!

Step 2: Start Small

Which do you think is easier: preparing three meals or just one? I'm sure you'd agree that planning and preparing one meal is much easier, which is exactly why starting small is so important. One big reason people fail to stick to a clean diet is because the idea of preparing three meals every single day overwhelms them. If you're just starting to improve your dietary habits, commit to making just *one* healthy meal per day. Then go about the rest of your day eating as you do right now, if you like. That will take a lot of the stress and pressure off and get you started.

Starting small is how I've helped thousands of people transform their health permanently. If you're a complete healthy-eating newbie—and even though I've got amazing recipes lined up for you in this cookbook—let's start at ground zero. I want you to start by focusing on just making one healthy meal. Nothing more, nothing less. The reason? It goes back to willpower. Your willpower is at its lowest at the end of the day (remember the battery analogy), so this is the time when most people make poor food choices because they don't want to think or put in effort. If you aren't sure what to make for dinner or are worried about finding the time, just choose any of the main dish, soup, or bowl recipes in this book and you'll be fine.

By starting small and focusing only on dinner, you'll have to think about 7 meals per week instead of 21 or more—much more manageable, right? Again, I would recommend this as an absolute beginner starting point. However, if you're ready and willing to jump right in to truly transform your body and health, then just follow the 10-Day Metabolic Reset in Chapter 13.

Step 3: Plan Ahead

Planning is critical to success in all areas of your life, especially when it comes to making your own food. If you get home after a long day and you don't know what you're having for dinner, you've already lost. Before you go to bed, you need to know what you're having for dinner tomorrow night. In fact, if you have a plan for the entire week, you'll be amazed at how much easier it is to make meals from scratch even after a long day. And that's because you've done the thinking ahead of time.

Here's how we're going to do this (assuming you're not following the 10-Day Metabolic Reset or even the 5-Day Food-Cycling Formula to the letter).

1. Sift through the pages in this cookbook and find the recipes that look the most appealing to you. Choose a variety of meals so you have breakfast, lunch, and dinner covered, if desired.

2. Now that you know what you're going to have, create a simple 7-day calendar and fill in your recipes at the various times of day you'll be eating them (breakfast, lunch, dinner, etc.).

3. Look at the recipes and jot down the exact groceries you need to make them happen. This is important so you're not aimlessly walking around the store grabbing random stuff you don't need. That's a huge mistake people make when they go grocery shopping. You should be like a laser-guided missile and know exactly what items you need.

If you don't want to bother with any of these three steps, then simply follow the 10-Day Metabolic Reset in Chapter 13 and you'll find every meal laid out for you in a way that coincides with my proven 5-Day Food-Cycling Formula for resetting your metabolism and burning fat. I hope the three steps I've covered in this chapter about setting up your environment to win, starting small, and planning ahead for success have struck a chord with you. These are very important steps to take to make any dietary plan work for you in the long run. And, speaking of the long run, healthy eating habits are what will keep you lean and healthy for good. So let's look at how to create healthy eating *habits* that actually stick using what I call my CPR Method.

Meg Loses 15 Pounds without Exercise

"I am 72 years old and have had a lifetime of ups and downs trying to lose weight, including surgery and wiring my mouth shut. I had been so depressed that last year I just gave up after eating 600 to 1,000 calories a day and not losing anything. I was tracking my food and weighing myself every day to no avail. I watched a free webinar that Yuri put on with several nutritionists and doctors, and it gave me hope because I didn't ever think about adding more good fats into my diet. When Yuri talked about his book, *The All-Day Fat-Burning Diet,* and the support group, I ordered it immediately. The recipes are wonderful. I have followed the plan for 5 weeks now and have lost 15 pounds without even doing any exercise. I have more energy to do more things during the day and my mood is happier. Love you, Yuri, and your devotion to helping others!"

How to Create Healthy Eating Habits That Actually Stick

Your life is a result of your habits. It's the little things you do, day in and day out, that truly make the biggest difference in time. And if, like so many other people I've helped over the years, you want to create healthy eating habits that actually stick, then I'm going to show you exactly how to do it with the proven CPR Method. I'll also debunk some of the biggest myths about habits so you can stop buying into them. But first, I want to share a few comments I see repeatedly from my clients, especially women. See if you can identify a common theme.

> "When I started the diet, I was severely addicted to sugar and wheat, but very quickly the cravings subsided. I felt I gained a control over my diet I had lacked for years. It felt more like a knot that was loosening, giving me a more relaxed relationship with food. I finally feel like I can hear my body telling me what it needs."

And this:

> "What you have provided me is control of my eating where I don't have to crave so much, and I also don't have to feel guilty if I don't eat so much. Being able to feel like I have control of my body is a wonderful change! I still have a few more pounds to go. I see this as a journey and look forward to learning more about what works best for me, my body, and my lifestyle."

And this:

> "I wanted to eat better, but I just resorted to my comfort food after every disappointment or failed attempt to do better. Food—especially sweets (chocolate is my *favorite*)—took me to my happy place. I knew I needed to change, but I honestly didn't know how."

Notice how *control* is a big focus here? It's ironic, because when creating healthy eating habits is the goal, self-control is actually the last thing you want to be focusing on. I'll show you why in a second, but let's understand how habits are formed in the first place.

How Habits Are Formed

Neuroscientists have traced our habit-making behaviors to a part of the brain called the basal ganglia, which also plays a key role in the development of emotions, memories, and pattern recognition. Decisions, meanwhile, take place in a different part of the brain called the prefrontal cortex. Why is this important? It's important because the goal of habit creation is to move the decision process from the prefrontal cortex to your basal ganglia. This is when a behavior truly becomes automatic—which is what we want.

To look at this another way, research shows that habit formation requires the following four stages of competency.

THE FOUR STAGES OF COMPETENCY

Stage 1: Unconscious Incompetence

You don't even know what you're not good at.

Stage 2: Conscious Incompetence

You're aware that you're not good at something.

Stage 3: Conscious Competence

You actively work to improve some behavior or skill. This is where you consciously work to improve. It requires heavy involvement of your prefrontal cortex.

Stage 4: Unconscious Competence

The behavior or skill has become automated (and instilled in your basal ganglia) and is no longer consciously controlled (by your prefrontal cortex).

When you first learn to drive, you're at Stage 1: You have no idea what's going on. But as you take your first few driving lessons and notice (consciously) that you are not that great at parallel parking, for instance, you move into Stage 2. However, with more practice, you move into Stage 3 and become a better parker (and driver), although it still requires a lot of focus and conscious attention.

With time and practice you (hopefully) reach the pinnacle—Stage 4—and can now parallel park while talking with a passenger or singing along to the radio. It's automatic. The process of creating healthy eating habits, or any other habit for that matter, follows a similar path. The goal is to make behavior automatic so that the decision-making part of your brain can shut down, which is a real advantage because it means you then have more mental energy to devote to something else. Creating healthy eating (and other) habits is all about moving a conscious behavior from your prefrontal cortex to your basal ganglia, where it is solidified and turned into an automatic routine. Next, let's look at how to do that.

The CPR Method

Of course, you don't physically touch parts of your brain to move stuff around; instead, a three-step process does the work for you. I call it the CPR Method, and it's the key to creating healthy eating habits that actually stick. I didn't invent this three-step process, although I believe I'm the first to name it. Credit for this "habit loop" discovery goes to Charles Duhigg, the author of *The Power of Habit*.[1]

In essence, all habits involve these three steps.

1. Cue (the trigger that initiates the behavior)
2. Practice or performance (the behavior itself)
3. Reward (the benefit you get from doing the behavior)

Duhigg calls them *cue, routine, reward*. (I think my wording is a little cleverer.) An important reminder: All behaviors reward you, even the not-so-good ones. The way our brains are wired makes it very challenging to create new healthy habits if we go about things without understanding this CPR framework. Smoking, using drugs, drinking, or eating sugar all have the same effect on the reward/pleasure center in our brain, known as the nucleus accumbens, which releases dopamine in the anticipation of a specific behavior (good or bad).

For example, here's what happens when you indulge in the habit of eating sugar.

1. You get stressed (cue).
2. You reach for a piece of chocolate (practice or performance).
3. You instantly feel calmer (reward).

See how primitive and simple that is? Repeat this over and over again and you've got a full-blown sugar/chocolate addiction (not a deficiency in magnesium, as some chocolate enthusiasts might proclaim). If you've got kids or live a stressful life (don't we all?), you can start to see how certain habits like grabbing a piece of chocolate or reaching for a glass of wine can easily spiral out of control. We all want to feel good. When we feel stressed, anxious, or upset, we'll do anything to return to our happy place, so keep in mind that attaching a positive reward to any behavior you want to turn into a lasting habit is very important.

Using the CPR Method to Create Healthier Eating Habits

Now that you know the three steps for creating a habit, here's how to structure the steps to create better eating habits that actually stick.

Step 1: Pick a Cue

As I'll show you in a moment, and as we discussed earlier, creating better eating habits has nothing to do with self-control or willpower. It's all about setting up your environment to support you. This is why the cue is such a critical part of forming new habits. A good cue does not rely on motivation, and it doesn't require you to remember to do your new habit. It simply makes it easy to start by piggybacking your new behavior onto something that you already do.

→ **Action Step** *Pick a cue by making a list of simple things you already do throughout the day: for instance, going to the bathroom, washing your face, tying your shoes, opening the fridge, and so forth. These are all every-day occurrences that require no thought and provide ideal "shuttles" on which to tie your desired behaviors.*

Three Ideas for Setting Up a Simple Cue for Better Eating Habits

Idea #1

Have a bowl of cut-up veggies (like bell peppers or cucumbers) easily accessible inside your fridge so that each time you open your fridge (the cue), you can quickly grab a healthy (and tiny) snack (the practice/performance).

Idea #2

Before going to bed, fill up a large glass of water and leave it on the counter in your kitchen. Then, first thing in the morning, when you enter your kitchen (the cue), drink your ready-made glass of water (practice/performance). To take things to the next level, refill your glass each time you drink it. Then, whenever you re-enter your kitchen, use that as your cue to drink a glass of water.

Idea #3

This idea requires my Energy Greens (which you can get at yurigreens.com). Instead of relying on coffee or sugar when you experience that midafternoon slump, let that slump in energy be your cue to add 1 tablespoon of your Energy Greens to a glass of water and drink it (practice/performance). Thus, whenever you feel tired, you condition yourself to reach for a healthy green elixir that takes 30 seconds to put together instead of relying on the short-lived reward (with long-term negative con-sequences) of caffeine or sugar.

Let me illustrate this with something everyone loves talking about: using the toilet. Flushing the toilet *after* the initial behavior of "doing your business" makes more sense than thinking that flushing the toilet first will prompt you to go to the bathroom. In the same way, you want to pair your new desired behavior with a prior cue. This is a consistent finding in the literature. One study found that those who flossed *after* brushing (rather than before) tended to form stronger flossing habits and, at their 8-month follow-up, had stronger habits and flossed more frequently.[2] In the toilet example above, going number one or number two would be the cue, and flushing would be the practice or performance. The reward is knowing that the smell of putrid waste won't permeate your entire house (a fun lesson to try to teach three young boys).

Step 2: Choose a Behavior That Is Almost Too Simple

How do you eat an elephant? One bite at a time. (I don't know who's eating elephants these days—hopefully no one.) The same thing applies to instilling healthy eating habits. Keep it super simple. Acclaimed Stanford professor of human behavior BJ Fogg recommends taking baby steps when thinking about your desired behaviors. He even advises creating "tiny habits" like brushing just *one* tooth at a time and building from there.[3] This has been shown to be much more effective at creating lasting habits than making monster resolutions like "I'm giving up gluten, dairy, and sugar all at the same time!" Start small and build from there.

⮕ **Action Step** *Decide what you want your new habit to be. Then ask yourself, "How can I make this new behavior so easy to do that I can't say no?"*

Step 3: Choose Your Reward(s)

I'm guilty of not celebrating my little and big victories as much as I should. However, it's an important practice I'm committed to doing every night before bed in my gratitude/success journal. Similarly, whenever *you* do your desired behavior, you need to celebrate it. This closes the feedback loop that tells your brain, "That behavior made me feel good. Let's do more of it."

In each of the ideas above for setting up a simple cue for better eating habits, the reward could be recognizing that you made a healthy food choice, which you can anchor with a fist pump and a mental or verbal "*Yes!*" Self-acknowledgment is a huge step in building your confidence and feeling better about yourself.

And, as I often say, "Great results come from feeling great." Plus, over time, you'll feel more energized, your clothes will fit better, and your health will improve, which will serve as ongoing rewards to keep you on track. Choose whatever reward you want (other than the very foods you're trying to move away from), but make sure it's meaningful to you.

How to Make Your Healthy Eating Habit Stick

With a new behavior under way, here are three simple action steps to make sure your healthy eating habit actually sticks.

Stick Strategy #1: Start with a super-small and easy-to-do behavior (as discussed above).

Stick Strategy #2: Increase your desired behavior each day, but in an incredibly small way.

Stick Strategy #3: Even after increasing your habit, keep repetitions super easy and break them down into easier pieces, if needed. (For example, if the idea of working out is overwhelming, just put on your tennis shoes. Then walk out the door. Then do one exercise, and so on.)

Let's look at the example of eating more green vegetables. After all, many people don't like eating green vegetables, so it could be a good place to start. And this dislike of greens is to be expected if you're used to eating processed food loaded with sugar, monosodium glutamate (MSG), salt, and other unhealthy ingredients that trick your palate and light up your brain's reward center. But here's how to make eating your greens an enjoyable and lasting habit, using the three stick strategies above.

1. On Day 1, take just *one* small bite of a leafy green vegetable. That's it. No harm done. Don't even make a salad. Just pull a piece of lettuce or kale (or other leafy green) out of the fridge and take a little bite.

2. On Day 2, do the same thing, but take *two* small bites of the green vegetable. *No más.*

3. Continue on this path until eating green vegetables becomes enjoyable and automatic. By this point, you'll probably be ready to actually make a salad and love every mouthful.

More Helpful Tips to Eat Healthier

Here are a few more ideas for how you can apply these three stick strategies to eat healthier on a consistent basis.

Drink More Water

- Take one small sip of water each time you enter your kitchen.

- On Day 2, take two sips of water each time you enter your kitchen.

- Keep adding more sips until you easily down a glass of water and actually look forward to it.

Get 8 to 10 Servings of Veggies and Fruit Each Day

First, cut up your favorite produce into bite-size pieces and keep them super easy to access in the fridge.

- On Day 1, each time you open the fridge, take just one piece.

- On Day 2, each time you open the fridge, take two pieces.

- Continue in this fashion and you'll be eating more veggies than a giraffe in no time.

Three Common Myths about Habits

Considering that so many people are conditioned to try to be "perfect," I think it's important to debunk three common myths about habits that could be holding you back. This is also the section where we'll dig a lot deeper into the false notion that willpower is required for eating well consistently (or successfully making any other change).

Myth #1:

It takes 21 days to create a habit

Sorry, not true. A lot of research has been done, and the reality is that some habits take much longer to develop than others. Dr. Phillippa Lally, a leading researcher in this area, found that it takes an average of 66 days for a behavior to become automatic and that the length of time that these behaviors stick is between 18 and 254 days and depends on the type of habit.[4]

For instance, simple behaviors (with less pain attached to them) like drinking water after lunch took only 56 days to stick, while doing situps every morning took 91 days in Dr. Lally's research. That length of time may sound slightly depressing, but just remember to keep the following pointers in mind.

Sciencia Loses 7 Pounds in 30 Days
While Going through Menopause

"All my life I have always been dieting and exercising but never consistently. I am 56 years old and going through menopause, and slowly the weight started creeping up on me. I was watching what I ate and exercising regularly to no avail. Then Yuri and his Fat Loss Summit came into my life, followed by the All-Day Fat-Burning Diet.

I really don't want to call it a diet because I am not counting calories. I am eating whole foods and absolutely delicious meals, not taking any diet supplements, *and* losing weight. I was 174 pounds when I started and I have lost 7 pounds in a month. I am getting great results on Yuri's eating plan. I am very grateful. Thanks, Yuri!"

- Take small steps. Don't try to do everything at once.
- Try to change only one habit at a time.
- Write down the habit you want to change, and write down specific plans for achieving that goal.
- Repeat the behavior you're aiming for as often as you can. The more a behavior is repeated, the more likely it will become instinctive.

This final tip leads to the next common myth.

Myth #2:
If you miss a day, you might as well start all over

Research has shown that skipping your habit once, no matter when, has no measurable impact on your long-term progress. Just get back on the horse and keep going. That's why I continue to remind you that progress, not perfection, is the goal. So please abandon the all-or-nothing mentality.

One really powerful technique I've used over the years to stay on track in many areas of my life is what I call "negative visualization." You've likely heard that you should only focus on what you want, because that's what you'll attract into your life. And while I agree with that, I also believe that foreseeing pitfalls and being prepared for them is just plain smart.

Negative visualization basically means having a plan B and plan C just in case plan A doesn't work out. The beauty of this is that you know how you would respond in advance, so there's no panic if the pitfall does occur. As a private pilot and lover of aviation, I can tell you that pilots relentlessly practice and prepare for worst-case scenarios. And thank goodness they do. Can you imagine if there was an in-flight electrical fire and the pilots had to scramble—at that point—to figure out a solution? If you apply the same thinking to your daily life, you can foresee potential obstacles and better prepare for them.

For example:

- You've got a company dinner next week. What challenges might arise that could derail you from your healthy-eating path? Figure out a solution now.

- You'll be traveling this weekend. So what will you eat on the road? Figure that out now.
- You're doing great and on the healthy-eating path, but all of a sudden you get some upsetting news that stresses you out. Will you turn to the chocolate and other de-stressing treats? Figure out a better alternative now.

You shouldn't expect to fail, but you should plan for failure. And even if you do fall off track, get right back on the next day. As you've undoubtedly experienced, good habits are a lot easier to form when you're riding the wave of momentum. Don't let the momentum swing back in the wrong direction.

Myth #3:
Creating new habits requires a lot of discipline and willpower

This is probably my favorite. The idea that willpower, self-control, and discipline are required to eat well is simply not true. It's the same reason why done-for-you meal plans and recipes are so important to have at your fingertips. They take the thinking out of food prep, especially after a long day when you're tired and low on willpower. Willpower is very much like a muscle that gets fatigued with constant use. One of the most famous studies on this topic, published in the *Journal of Personality and Social Psychology* back in 1998, examined the effect of a tempting food challenge designed to deplete participants' willpower through the awful power of an unfulfilled promise of chocolate![5]

In the first part of the trial, the researchers kept the participants in a room that smelled of freshly baked chocolate cookies. Then they teased them by showing them the actual treats alongside other chocolate-flavored confections. While some test subjects got to indulge their sweet tooth, those whose willpower was being tested in the experimental condition were asked to eat radishes instead. How cruel.

After the initial food bait and switch, the participants were asked to complete a puzzle, which really tested their persistence (or resolve). The effect of the food manipulation was undeniable. Those who ate radishes made far fewer attempts at the puzzle and gave up more than *twice* as fast as the chocolate-eating participants. In other words, those who had to resist the sweets and force themselves to eat the radishes could no longer find the will to fully engage in another torturous task. They were already too tired.[6]

The key finding from this seemingly silly study was a breakthrough: Self-control and willpower are fleeting strengths that are used up across different sorts of tasks (decision making, resisting temptation, heavy mental work, etc.). And they are depleted like a smartphone battery after constant use. The pivotal study prompted 1,282 future studies involving everything from consumer to criminal behavior. For instance, another famous study on court hearings found that at the beginning of the day, a judge was likely to give a favorable ruling about 65 percent of the time. However, as the morning wore on and the judge became drained from making more and more decisions, the likelihood of a criminal getting a favorable ruling steadily dropped to *zero*! After taking a lunch break, however, the judge returned to the courtroom refreshed, and the likelihood of a favorable ruling immediately jumped back up to 65 percent. And then, as the hours moved on, the percentage of favorable rulings would fall back down to zero by the end of the day.[7] (So, the take-home message is to fight those parking or speeding tickets early in the day or just after lunch.)

The Interesting Relationship between Stress, Blood Sugar, and Self-Control

Another important finding from the radish and chocolate study is that willpower seems to be tied to our blood glucose, suggesting that willpower can be negatively affected during times of low blood sugar. This is why self-control can deteriorate during premenstrual syndrome (ladies, think chocolate cravings) and during periods of low food intake, especially if you suffer from hypoglycemia. That's why people may become cranky and irritable when they have low blood sugar and are hungry—something many call "hangry."

Another article published in the journal *Personality and Social Psychology Review* suggests blood glucose is one important part of the energy source for better self-control, and the more we use our self-control and willpower, the quicker we deplete large amounts of glucose.[8] Perhaps you've had days when you've gotten home from work exhausted, maybe not physically, but mentally.

And that was likely due to all the decisions you made, restraint you employed, and mental work you did during the day. Well, depleted willpower at night usually means "finger cooking" (aka dialing for take-out or delivery). After all, it's so much easier to order take-out than to spend even 15 minutes preparing a meal. That's why you have to set up your environment to win.

You know you can't rely on sheer determination or willpower to eat well consistently. And we know that dinnertime is the weak point for most of us, when even the best of intentions can quickly go awry. Therefore, the key to healthy eating habits—aside from the habit strategies we've discussed above—is to set up your environment to support you in your weakest moments. Here are a few ways to do that, some of which recap what we discussed earlier in this chapter.

- **Make sure your kitchen is squeaky clean** (instead of cluttered) so you can think a little more clearly in moments of weakness. After all, a cluttered surrounding leads to a cluttered mind, which gravitates toward seeking escape or a quick-fix meal or treat.

- **Follow a meal plan** so you know exactly what you're having for your next meal—ahead of time, no thinking required. Don't wait until you're hangry to decide what to eat—that's a recipe for disaster. Use Chapter 13, The 10-Day Metabolic Reset, for ultimate convenience.

- **Have all the necessary ingredients on hand and easily accessible.** If you have to go to the store at the last minute, your chances of making a healthy choice drop even further. Remember, make good behavior very easy, which means having the right foods at your fingertips.

- **Throw out the junk.** We all know it's easier to reach into a bag of potato chips than it is to make a healthy meal, even one that takes just a few minutes. Your goal should be to make healthy choices very accessible and unhealthy choices extremely inaccessible. The easiest way is to simply throw out the junk food altogether.

Habits are vital to every aspect of your life. I hope you take away that even big changes should begin with super-small microcommitments. Make a mountain a molehill, and you'll be much more likely to create healthy eating habits that last for good. Now it's time to look at how to prepare your fat-burning kitchen. Are you excited?

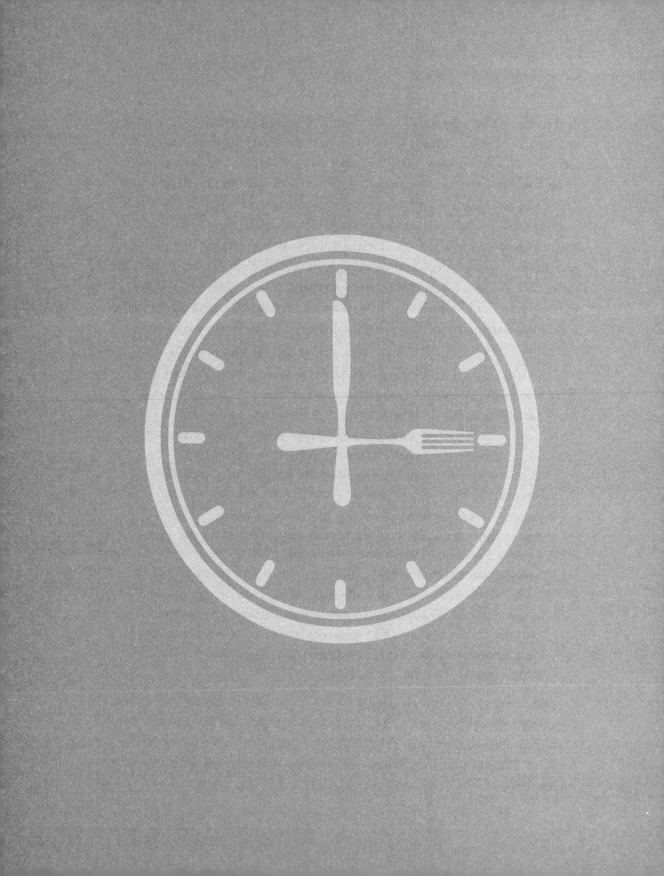

Chapter 3

Preparing Your Fat-Burning Kitchen

FAIL TO PLAN AND YOU PLAN TO FAIL. That's what they say, right? It's absolutely true. As a highly motivated action taker, I've realized that every hour of planning saves you a dozen more in poorly executed action. This chapter will help you plan and prepare for ultimate success. You'll discover which foods to eat and why they're so good for you, which foods to avoid, and how to get your cooking tools in order so you can feel like a hero in your kitchen as you whip these recipes together.

Kitchen Must-Haves

Before we dive mouth-first into the delicious recipes in this cookbook, it might be helpful to know what tools and basic kitchen cookware you'll need to make them. Thankfully, it's a pretty short list, and I bet you probably already have most of these items. So before I walk you through some of the food staples to have on hand and explain why they're good for you and so helpful at burning fat, let's first go through the tools you need to prepare the recipes.

Pots and Pans

A good set of skillets (or frying pans) and pots is essential to any healthy kitchen. I like skillets that have some depth so you can also use them as a wok for stir-fries. I'm assuming you already have a set of pots and pans, but if you're in the market for a new one, I'll give you some pointers on the best ones to choose, from a health perspective.

In general, I recommend staying away from Teflon and other nonstick cookware because it often leaches chemicals into your food. Instead, your best bet is to go with stainless steel, with enameled cast iron as a second option. Stainless steel cookware is beneficial because it's nonreactive (meaning you can cook any kind of food in it without chemical leaching), heavy, durable, dishwasher-safe, and relatively inexpensive.

The main downside is that it usually has poor heat transfer and distribution, but you can solve this problem by buying better-quality (and higher-priced) stainless steel cookware with an added inner core made of copper or aluminum, which improves the heat conductivity. Since the aluminum or copper is sandwiched between layers of steel and does not come in contact with the food, these types of stainless steel cookware are fine to use. All-Clad is a great example of high-end stainless steel cookware. However, enameled cast iron can be a good option for a Dutch oven. It is durable, nonreactive, naturally nonstick if properly seasoned, easy to clean, and distributes heat evenly and retains heat well, making it great for long, low simmering and browning. Popular enameled cast-iron brands include Le Creuset and Staub.

A Good Set of Knives

Although you won't need all of the following knives for the recipes in this book, a good basic knife set should include:

- An all-purpose utility knife (5 inches)—used for a range of purposes; often a good choice for your first knife, as it can do many things.
- A chef's knife (7.8 to 9 inches)—used for chopping, dicing, mincing, and cutting. You will use this knife often for these recipes.
- A vegetable or paring knife (3 inches)—used for peeling, cutting, and trimming small food items that you hold in your hand (such as trimming small potatoes). You'll also use this knife often in these recipes.
- A cleaver—used for meat, with a smaller version for chopping herbs, etc. Buy a cleaver only if you need to chop serious pieces of meat.
- A carving knife—used for getting thin and even slices of meat from roasts, roasted poultry, etc. Great for Thanksgiving but rarely used otherwise.
- Sharpening steel, knife-honing stone, or electric honer.

There are several considerations when choosing a knife, including weight, balance, and blade material. A lightweight knife is good for speed and precision, whereas a heavy knife requires far more work when chopping a lot of light ingredients. However, a heavier knife is better for chopping foods such as nuts, fresh ginger, and other harder ingredients.

Quality knives tend to have very good balance, with not too much weight in either the blade or the handle. The way to test is to place your finger at the finger grip where the blade meets the handle, holding the knife horizontally with the cutting edge down. A quality, well-balanced knife will balance at that point and not fall off your finger—it is essentially the leverage point.

Chopping, Dicing, Julienning, and Mincing: What's the Difference?

Throughout this cookbook (and others) you'll see recommendations for certain ingredients to be chopped, diced, julienned, or minced. Here, I'll walk you through the differences.

- *Chopped* usually refers to cutting a vegetable or other food item into ¾-inch squares, as when cutting something large (think potatoes, quartered onions, melon) into small chunks.

- *Diced* refers to cutting an ingredient into ¼-inch cubes. A lot of recipes start with a base of sautéed diced celery, carrots, onions, or bell peppers.

- *Julienned* refers to cutting vegetables, etc., into long matchsticks that have a thickness of approximately ⅛ inch. Bell peppers or even French fries might be julienned.

- *Minced* means chopping ingredients into as small dice as you can, usually ¹⁄₁₆ inch. Garlic is the most commonly minced ingredient.

The key reason to consider balance is that a well-balanced knife makes any cutting action easier and more effortless. If you are planning on using the knife for large quantities of ingredients, a balanced knife will impose far less strain on your arm. Good knives are often made of nonstainless steel (carbon steel), which can be sharpened to a good edge fairly quickly, but be sure to store them in a knife block so they do not rust.

Cutting Board

This is pretty straightforward, as you'll need a good surface on which to chop your ingredients. I recommend bamboo cutting boards. Even the hardest of wood cutting boards will be scarred by repeated cutting and chopping, which will leave pockets for moisture, food particles, and bacteria to accumulate. Bamboo, on the other hand, is often dense enough to resist knife scarring and naturally resists water penetration, which prevents bacteria from finding a place to form.

Spiralizer

A spiralizer is an inexpensive tool that turns fresh veggies, most often zucchini, into faux noodles (zoodles, if you will). It's a great tool to have on hand for making raw pastas instead of relying on traditional (and slightly heavier) wheat- or gluten-free pasta noodles. Several of the recipes in this cookbook (see Zippy Zoodles on page 166) call for a spiralizer. If you don't have one, you can always use a vegetable peeler.

Vegetable Peeler

If you can't get your hands on a spiralizer, then you can always rely on a vegetable peeler to make your zucchini noodles, although they'll be more like fettuccine than spaghetti noodles. A vegetable peeler also comes in handy for peeling many of the root vegetables called for throughout the cookbook.

Blender

Smoothies, soups, sauces, and more—a good blender can make all of them. I am a big fan of the Vitamix. Sure, it's about $400, but I've had mine for 10 years. That's a pretty good investment, if you ask me. Nonetheless, even a $50 blender will be able to handle all of the necessary blending chores in this cookbook.

Food Processor

Although a good blender can often do the job of a food processor, I like having both. I use my food processor to accelerate chopping, especially of nuts, and for making dips like hummus. Again, it's not required, only recommended. If a recipe calls for a food processor and you don't have one, just use a blender (at low speed) instead.

All-Day Fat-Burning "Clean and Lean" Foods

Although these foods were covered in detail in *The All-Day Fat-Burning Diet*, I'd like to go over them briefly with you here again. After all, maybe you didn't read the first book, yet you should still know about these important fat-burning foods. While reading, keep in mind that every food on the planet contains fat, protein, and carbohydrate in addition to hundreds of smaller micronutrients. Thus, it's not completely accurate to classify one food as just "fat" and another as "protein." For our purposes, however, I've put the foods into each category based on their predominant macronutrient. For instance, certain high-fat nuts are in the Fit Fats group, while other high-protein nuts are listed as Clean Proteins.

Fit Fats

Let's get one thing straight: Fat is not the enemy. Healthy fats are extremely good for you and needed for proper cellular health, hormone production, and so much more. A diet lacking in good fats is like eating cake without icing: It's just not the same. The *wrong* fats are the bigger issue. The reason is because the most commonly used fats and oils these days are highly inflammatory and often rancid vegetable oils like canola oil, soybean oil, and many others, as you'll see in a second. With that said, please remember that most of the best sources of healthy Fit Fats are also vegetable based. So let me clear the air here.

Vegetable oils (and margarine, made from these oils) are oils extracted from seeds like rapeseed (canola oil), soybeans (soybean oil), corn (corn oil), sunflower seeds (sunflower oil), safflower seeds (safflower oil), and so on. Interestingly, these oils were not a part of the human diet until the early 1900s, when new chemical processes allowed them to be extracted. The trouble begins with the fact that, unlike coconut oil, these vegetable oils can't be extracted just by pressing or naturally separating them from the seed. Instead, they must be chemically removed, deodorized, and altered. And herein lies the problem: Vegetable oils are highly susceptible to damage from heat, oxygen, and light. This is because they are polyunsaturated fats (meaning they have more than one double bond and are liquid at room temperature) and their chemical structure is highly volatile.

Butter and coconut oil are very stable saturated fats. Their chemical "chains" are more resilient to exposure to heat, oxygen, and light, which is why they are very good options to use when cooking or baking. Liquid vegetable oils, on the other hand—even healthy ones like olive and flaxseed—get damaged when exposed to the three aforementioned elements and therefore should never be heated, let alone subjected to intense processing.

And that brings us back to the most common vegetable oils in today's foods—the ones you see listed on the back of almost every packaged food: canola oil, corn oil, and soybean oil. The problem is that these polyunsaturated fats are highly unstable (as previously mentioned) and oxidize easily, and this oxidization causes serious inflammation inside the body. And we know what inflammation does to our chances of losing weight, right? Aside from being oxidized and having turned rancid from intense processing en route to store shelves, most of these vegetable oils are also very high in inflammatory omega-6 fatty acids. You may have heard of omega-3s and -6s; well, there's a big difference between the two. The former is highly anti-inflammatory and thus very good for your body, whereas the latter is the complete opposite.

Ideally, the human body needs omega-3 and omega-6 fats in balance, preferably in a 1:2 ratio. However, the modern American diet is closer to 1:20. This means that, in general, we are consuming 10 times more inflammatory oils than anti-inflammatory ones. Let's put a stop to that right now and focus on only consuming good-quality Fit Fats. By doing so, you help lower inflammation in your body, which in turn helps release stubborn fat more effortlessly while improving many aspects of your health.

Fit Fats include healthy fats that are saturated (such as butter and coconut oil), monounsaturated (olives, avocados), and polyunsaturated (flaxseed and fish oil). These fats provide vital building blocks that improve the quality of your cell mem-

Avocados as Sunscreen?

You may be aware that avocado consumption has a protective effect on your cardio-vascular system. Yes, good fat is good for you. But did you know that avocados contain polyhydroxylated fatty alcohols that have been shown to suppress the inflammatory response and provide sunscreenlike protection against UV-induced damage?[1] Well, now you do. Maybe that's why they're so popular in hot climates. Half an avocado per day (or more if you like) is all you need to enjoy all of its health benefits.

branes (which is partially reflected in the quality of your skin, hair, and nails), serve as an important building block for your hormones, provide the building blocks for the myelin sheath around your nerves, and so much more.

This chart provides an overview of the Fit Fats and Filthy Fats. Note that foods are placed in each category based on their dominant type of fat, since most foods contain varying levels of all three types of fat. Throughout the recipes in this book, you'll find a healthy dose of most of these Fit Fats.

FIT FATS (ENJOY THESE)			FILTHY FATS (AVOID THESE)
Saturated	Monounsaturated	Polyunsaturated	Polyunsaturated
Coconut oil	Avocados	Algae oil	Canola oil
Ghee	Brazil nuts	Fish oil	Corn oil
Grass-fed butter	Macadamia nuts (and macadamia nut oil)	Flaxseed oil	Cottonseed oil
	Olives (and olive oil)	Hemp seed oil	Grapeseed oil
		Sunflower seeds	Margarine
		Walnuts	Peanut oil
			Safflower oil
			Shortening
			Soybean oil
			Sunflower oil

Clean Proteins

I'll talk about the fat-burning importance of protein in the next section. Here, I want to encourage you to get more of your protein from plant-based sources. There are many myths about plant proteins, but just know that you can easily meet all of your protein needs through quality plant-based foods. Plant-based proteins are less acidic and usually contain a greater array of nutrients than their animal counterparts. The only dilemma with plant proteins is that they also come with more carbohydrates. For the most part, that's not a problem, but when the program calls for you to eat fewer carbs than usual—like on your Low-Carb Days—you'll want to cut back a bit.

If you're not fully vegan, then you'll be happy to know that there are also many animal-based dishes in this book. If you're eating animal products, then please do your best to get organic, wild, free-range, or grass-fed sources whenever possible. You are what you eat (and absorb), so you don't want to be ingesting consistent amounts of bioaccumulated pesticides, hormones, antibiotics, or other artificial ingredients in the "feed" these animals have been forced to live on. After all, most commercially raised animals are pumped full of hormones and antibiotics and fed unnatural foods like soy and grains, which degrade their health and end up adding to your body's toxic load.

The following chart lays out the Clean Proteins, along with examples of those you should avoid.

CLEAN PROTEINS (ENJOY THESE)		DIRTY PROTEINS (AVOID THESE)	
Plant-Based	Animal (organic, free range, grass fed, wild)	Plant-Based	Animal
Almonds (raw or soaked)	Anchovies	Soy	Any products from conventionally raised farm animals
Black beans*	Bacon (nitrate-free)		Fast-food meat
Cannellini beans*	Beef		Hot dogs
Chickpeas (garbanzo beans)*	Chicken		
	Crab		
Hemp seeds	Eggs		
Kidney beans*	Game (bison, etc.)		
Lentils (cooked or sprouted)*	Ham (nitrate-free)		
	Lamb		
Navy beans*	Lobster		
Pinto beans*	Oysters		
	Pork		
	Salmon (wild caught)		
	Sardines		
	Shrimp		
	Trout, rainbow		
	Turkey		

*Indicates a higher presence of starchy carbs in addition to its protein content.

Starchy Carbs and Fruit

I don't think I did this section justice in the previous book, so I'm going to spend a bit of time explaining why starchy carbs and fruit are helpful and important for your ability to lose weight. But before I dive into that, these are the healthy starchy carbs and fruits that I recommend. Obviously, you would avoid these on your Low-Carb Days.

STARCHY CARBS AND FRUIT (ENJOY THESE)			REFINED, FATTENING CARBS (AVOID THESE)
Starchy Carbs	Fruit	Nonglutinous Grains	
Beets	Apples	Amaranth	Candy
Carrots	Bananas	Buckwheat	Chips
Parsnips	Berries (all types)	Gluten-free oats	French fries
Potatoes (ideally cooked, then cooled)	Cucumbers	Millet	Nonorganic dried fruit
	Dried fruit (organic)	Quinoa	Packaged cereals
Sweet potatoes	Figs		Pastries
Turnips	Grapefruit		Pizza
Yams	Grapes		Rye bread
	Lemon		Wheat-based breads
	Mango		Wheat-based pastas
	Melon (all types)		
	Oranges		
	Papaya		
	Pears		
	Pineapple		
	Tomatoes		

→ **Did You Know?** *The bananas you see at the grocery store are all genetically identical, because they come from trees that have been cloned for decades. Ever notice how all bananas seem to look the same, even though other fruits (like apples) have many different varieties? That's because only bananas of the Cavendish variety are sold in stores. And while there are* *indeed many species in the banana genus, fruit corporations long ago decided that it would best serve their profits to train consumers to expect all bananas to be identical. In order to preserve their distinctive properties, Cavendish bananas are never allowed to reproduce. This means they all have the exact same genetic code as the first Cavendish tree selected by United Fruit Corporation in the 1950s. Another fun fact: Bananas are also the only fruit to grow upside down. Pretty cool.*

Since many people have asked me about sweeteners, here's a list of All-Day Fat-Burning–approved sweeteners and ones to stay away from. Please bear in mind that just because many of these are approved doesn't mean you should consume them in large quantities. A little here and there is best.

SWEETENERS			
Best	Better	Good (in very small amounts)	Avoid
Erythritol	Maple syrup	Brown sugar	Acesulfame potassium
Stevia	Raw honey	Coconut sugar	Agave
Xylitol	Sugar alcohols (sorbitol, maltitol, etc.)		Aspartame
			Glucose-fructose (sugar), high-fructose corn syrup
			Sucralose
			White sugar

→ Did You Know? *High-fructose corn syrup, found in many foods, is made using a toxic chemical catalyst, and most HFCS products may even be tainted with mercury. HFCS is used as a sweetener in nearly all mainstream packaged foods in the United States, from bread to soda and even breakfast cereal. It has been blamed for increasing the number of empty calories in the US diet, and researchers have linked it to diabetes and obesity.[2] Another danger from this common sugar swap comes from the toxic chemicals that are used to turn corn into cornstarch and then into HFCS. One of these chemicals,*

glutaraldehyde, is so dangerous that small quantities can cause damage to the
stomach lining. Like other chemical disinfectants, it can irritate the lungs,
eyes, and throat and can cause headaches or dizziness if inhaled. Just another
reason to eat real food and avoid the chemical, man-made nonsense.[3]

Why Carbs Are Good

Let's get back to our discussion on carbs. When used strategically, they are very helpful (and important) for your ability to lose weight. If you go too low carb for too long, your body will crash and you'll eventually rebel by going on a carb binge. Plus, no one feels good when they've restricted their carb intake for long periods of time, even if they are eating higher amounts of healthy fats. That's why this is not a low-carb diet.

Without going too deep into the science of why strategically eating more carbohydrates is good for you, here's a quick overview.

- It prevents thyroid function from plummeting, which is important for keeping your metabolic rate highly active to help you burn fat.
- It helps prevent hypothalamic amenorrhea in women, a starvation-related response that impairs normal hormone function, which can result in increased body fat, lower bone density, and impaired fertility.
- It maintains testosterone levels and prevents cortisol from increasing due to extended periods of low caloric intake, which helps prevent muscle loss and thus metabolic decline.
- It helps to ensure optimal levels of leptin, the hormone that tells your brain you're full, which prevents you from overeating. Conversely, with caloric restriction, leptin levels fall and you end up bingeing because your brain believes you are starving.

As you can see, carbohydrates play multiple important roles in your body, so they're not something you can simply go without. Choosing to go low carb indefinitely is certainly an option, and you will likely lose a lot of weight, but there's a strong chance you'll end up feeling pretty miserable in the process and regain any lost weight if you choose to introduce carbs back into your diet. Instead, by following the 5-Day Food-Cycling Formula that *The All-Day Fat-Burning Diet* and this cookbook are based on, you can enjoy the right carbs at the right times and shed weight safely and sustainably.

Carb Timing

We've been led to believe that eating carbs for breakfast is the best way to start the day. You can thank big cereal companies for this idea, since it's really their decades of marketing that have brainwashed our culture into thinking that cereal, bagels, muffins, and other carbs are the way to start the day. In fact, walk into any Starbucks and good luck finding any food item that isn't a refined carbohydrate (think pastries) that will skyrocket your blood sugar and leave you feeling like a zombie about an hour later.

Here's what you need to know: If you have carbohydrates for breakfast, they're going to blunt your body's natural cortisol response, which is highest in the morning. This is because cortisol naturally breaks down glycogen stores in your body into readily accessible blood sugar. Therefore, if you eat a lot of carbs in the morning, you'll be giving yourself an influx of blood sugar. This means that cortisol doesn't have to do its job, and you'll end up with a lower cortisol response in the morning.

I know what you're thinking: "Cortisol is bad, right?" The truth is, cortisol isn't inherently bad. It all depends on how much of it you have in your body—too much is a very bad thing—and when it's present. Cortisol is an important part of your natural biology and has a natural rhythm throughout the day: highest in the morning, lowest at night. If we do things to offset that, we're going to start running into problems over time. That's one of the reasons why eating carbohydrates in the morning is not the best idea.

Furthermore, early-morning carb consumption makes you feel sluggish because carb intake (especially of refined carbs) spikes your blood sugar. As a result, insulin is released to remove the excess sugar out of the blood and into storage. When this happens, most people experience a significant drop in blood sugar that leaves them feeling "hangry," or even like a zombie: They get anxious, have trouble focusing, and can only think about getting their next sugar fix to come back to life. That's no way to start your day, wouldn't you agree?

That's why my advice is to have more of your carbohydrates later in the day and have more protein in the morning. You can still have your green juice or smoothie if you like, but get some protein in there as well—it's going to keep you full longer and mentally sharper. You can still have a steak and salad for dinner if you want—I'm not saying you can't—but do not be afraid of carbohydrates.

Evelyn's Now 15 Pounds Lighter and Has More Mental Clarity and Energy

"If someone would have told me 3 months ago that soon I'd no longer be drinking caffeine, eating dairy, and I'd be gluten-free, I'd have said they were crazy! Initially, I feared the All-Day Fat-Burning Diet would be painfully restrictive, but it wasn't! I did struggle with headaches and feeling like I had a brain fog as I detoxed from caffeine, gluten, and dairy. But after a few days my brain felt clearer and the headaches were gone.

"I was worried about the 5-day food cycle, fearing that I might be hungry or find the food unpalatable. But I found the meals to be delicious, and each evening I was excited to see what new dishes were on the menu for the next day. Creamy kale salad, Thai salad, and cooled potatoes are a few of my favorite meals. I was never hungry and was surprised to find I had very few cravings.

"What I really liked about this plan is that it's real food and there is no calorie counting. I love cooking, and following this plan allows me to continue to enjoy that. It has introduced me to new food combinations and encouraged me to really listen to the needs of my body. I've lost 15 pounds, feel mentally clearer, and have lots of energy. I look forward to continuing on this new lifestyle. With the support of Yuri Elkaim and the Facebook support group, I know I'll be successful."

Mind you, this doesn't mean I'm advocating for you to have a slice of chocolate cake each night before bed. What I am saying is that having carbohydrates later in the day is better for your body's innate circadian rhythm, which is going to help you lose weight and stay lean. Plus, eating carbs later in the day actually helps you sleep better, because when you bring carbohydrates in, the level of free tryptophan in your blood increases. Tryptophan then crosses into the brain, where it can be converted into serotonin, which is a relaxing neurotransmitter. Finally, serotonin is converted into melatonin, which is the neurotransmitter/ hormone that allows your body to fall asleep.

I know this is very technical, but just remember this: Eating more of your carbohydrates later in the day won't make you fat but will help you lose fat (by honoring your natural body rhythms) and sleep better. I hope this gives you some clarity on the right approach to eating carbs. You don't have to stay away from them, but knowing exactly when to eat carbs will do wonders for your health!

Four Odd Carbs for Faster Fat Loss (and Better Health)

By now, you either think I'm crazy for all this carb talk or you're happy that I'm finally making sense of mystical carbs, once and for all. Good carbs: Who would've thought such a thing could exist? Given that carbs are demonized as the cause of all weight gain in most fitness circles these days, I completely understand if you're suspicious of the term *good carbs*, but it's true: There are good carbs out there that don't make you put on weight. In fact, these good carbs help you burn fat.

It's all about eating the right good carbs strategically throughout the week— hence our 5-Day Food-Cycling Formula. Here, I'd like to share four of my favorite carbs for burning fat and improving your overall health. You might be surprised by some of them. Keep in mind that, as good as they are for you, I still recommend that you avoid them on your Low-Carb Days (which is just once per week) in order to keep your net carb count down.

Bananas

Bananas get a lot of flack for being extra sweet and a source of a lot of sugar. And that is true if you eat them when they're overly ripe. The secret is all in how you eat them. As bananas ripen, they become more yellow, with dark blotches on them. When this happens, their natural levels of sugar increase. However, when a banana is unripe, it contains a higher amount of a specific type of carbohydrate called resistant starch that does not get digested and absorbed by your body, which means it doesn't impact your blood sugar in a negative way.

The other great thing about resistant starch is that it acts as food for the good bacteria in your gut. And one of the by-products of the breakdown of resistant starch by your gut bacteria is butyric acid. Butyric acid, if you're wondering, is one of the most important short-chain fatty acids for healing your gut.

Why does that matter? Because your gut is really your body's second brain, and it's intricately linked to your immune system. Remember all that inflammation we talked about being bad for your body and halting your fat loss? It's stimulated or thwarted at the level of your gut and the immune cells surrounding your gut. The healthier your gut, the less troublesome food particles can seep into your bloodstream and trigger unwanted inflammation.

To improve the health of your gut, you can't just rely on probiotics. You also need to feed those good bacteria with their ideal food, which is resistant starch (and other fibers). Unripened bananas, with their high levels of resistant starch, are a great source of food for those good bacteria that doesn't impact your belly, your waistline, or your blood sugar in any way.

Cooked-and-Cooled Potatoes

This is probably a shocker. Yes, white potatoes are good carbs. Yes, you can eat them. The thing is, you shouldn't eat them as you normally would. For example, if you cook them and mash them up, they're generally higher glycemic, meaning they're going to spike your blood sugar and lead to fat storage. They aren't the best thing for diabetics (or anyone interested in losing weight) to be eating. However, if you cook them and put them in the fridge to cool, what happens is an

Need More Proof That Resistant Starch Is Good for You?

Research from the journal *Diabetes Care* showed that sneaking just 5 grams of this superstarch into a daily muffin helped overweight subjects lower and stabilize their blood sugar levels much more effectively than those who did not receive the super-starch.[4] Since sugary, wheat-loaded muffins are notoriously bad for diabetics (and most people, in general), these results are nothing short of amazing. A 2005 study in the *American Journal of Clinical Nutrition* showed that adding just a few table-spoons of this superstarch improved insulin sensitivity by 33 percent after just 4 weeks![5]

Studies also showed that resistant starch reduces abdominal fat by more than simply diluting the number of calories eaten. It's been theorized that it affects energy balance through a signaling mechanism involving the activation of satiety hormones, gut hormones peptide YY (PYY) and glucagon-like peptide 1 (GLP-1), by short-chain fatty acids (namely butyrate) that are produced in the gut by fermenting resistant starch. One study revealed that adding resistant starch to the diet over just 12 weeks led to a 50 percent drop in abdominal fat compared to the control group.[6]

expansion of resistant starch inside the potato. There it is again, that resistant starch. Notice a pattern?

If you're wondering how you can pull this off and enjoy those potatoes, look no further than some of the potato salads in this cookbook. If you're willing to try something a little different, you can also use raw or unmodified potato starch, which you can find in your health food store. Mind you, it's not the same as potato flour. It's actually quite different. To make good use of it, you want to add a tablespoon to a glass of water or your smoothie, and that's it. Although none of the smoothie recipes in this cookbook explicitly list raw potato starch as an ingredient, it is certainly a tasteless upgrade you can incorporate into any of them.

If you feel a little bit of gastric distress, that's okay, that's normal. It takes a week or two for your gut to readjust and get used to these prebiotics that are very, very good for you. Most of us don't get enough fiber or these types of prebiotics, so when we start eating them, our body goes into a bit of shock. If this happens, lower the dose, and increase it slowly.

If you haven't figured it out by now, gut health and weight loss are intertwined. That's why a healthy dose of good bacteria in your gut and the right food to support it are massively important for helping you lose fat and improve your overall health.

Berries

Anything that ends in *-berry* is good for your health and your waistline. You can throw cherries in there as well. What makes them so amazing? Berries and cherries are fruits with a very low glycemic index, so they're not going to spike your blood sugar, and if your blood sugar doesn't get spiked, then insulin is not going to be released in high quantities. This is good because insulin is a storage hormone, and too much of it will take the sugar out of your blood and store it in your fat cells. As you might imagine, that's not a very good thing. Plus, high levels of insulin trigger inflammation in the body. Not good.

Anything you can do to mitigate insulin's response will be very helpful for your ability to lose weight and keep it off. That's why berries are one of my top fat-burning foods. Plus, studies have suggested that the consumption of

Blueberries for Better Blood Sugar Levels

Blueberries are loaded with disease-fighting antioxidants, but they're also tremendously good at stabilizing your blood sugar. This is extremely important for diabetics and fat-loss seekers alike, since rises in blood sugar and insulin (normally seen after eating high-sugar foods) prevent your body from burning fat. In one study on individuals diagnosed with type 2 diabetes, study participants who consumed at least three servings of low-GI fruits per day (including blueberries) saw significant improvement in their regulation of blood sugar over a 3-month period of time.[7] Blueberries also provide a very good amount of fiber (nearly 4 grams per cup), which helps to explain why they're so beneficial for keeping your blood sugar levels and waistline in check.

blueberries provides several health benefits, including improvement in cognitive function, antioxidant effects, protection against inflammation, and modulation of obesity and adiposity.[8, 9, 10] So enjoy blueberries (and other berries) to your heart's content.

Legumes

You'll find many recipes in this book that incorporate legumes like lentils, beans, and chickpeas. If you have a problem with legumes (and I'm talking to you die-hard paleo fans out there), then you can either skip those recipes or reconsider why you're avoiding them in the first place. There is way too much research showing the benefits of regular legume consumption to completely eradicate them from your diet.

I'm here to inform you that the anti-bean brigade has it all wrong. Yes, legumes may make you a bit gassy or upset your tummy sometimes, but as with resistant starch, there's a good amount of fiber in there—oligosaccharides and stuff like that—that your body's not necessarily used to. With time and regular consumption, that gas and bloating will go away, if they even occur in the first place.

Research conclusively shows that an increased intake of legumes and beans decreases our risk of cardiovascular disease. You might be surprised to learn that a 2014 meta-analysis in the *American Journal of Clinical Nutrition* found that legume consumption was inversely related with heart disease among the 501,791 individuals studied. Basically, eating more legumes lowered people's risk of heart attack.[11] Another 2014 review of the literature set out to examine the effect of legume intake on markers of inflammation in the body, including C-reactive protein. The researchers compiled all the studies on the topic and found that legume consumption contributes to reductions in C-reactive protein concentrations, which means less deadly and fat-inducing inflammation in the body![12]

But what about weight loss? Does legume consumption directly help you shed some of those extra pounds? You bet. These findings have been supported by research like a 2011 study in the *European Journal of Nutrition* in which overweight and obese subjects were randomly assigned to either a calorie-restricted, legume-free diet (the control group) or a calorie-restricted, legume-based diet (the legume group) for 8 weeks. The legume group was asked to eat only four weekly servings (160 to 235 grams total per week) of lentils, chickpeas, peas, or beans in addition to their regular food. At the end of the 8-week study, the legume group saw significant reductions in inflammatory markers, such as C-reactive protein. They also lost more weight and benefited from significant improvements in blood lipid profiles and blood pressure, compared with the control group.[13]

So eating legumes decreases your risk of heart disease, reduces inflammation, and directly helps you lose weight. Why on earth would you demonize such an important food group? Plus, for vegans and meat-eaters alike, legumes are an incredible source of protein (about 16 grams per cup) and have high levels of fiber—something you don't get by deriving all your protein from meat. The other thing I love about legumes is that they're so versatile. You can add them to a soup, stew, or chili, eat them on their own, or have them as a side. They're a tremendous food type, and you should be eating more of them.

I hope this section has helped you see the light on good carbs. Not all carbohydrates are evil, and the ones I've listed certainly won't make you gain weight. They'll actually help you lose it and improve your health in the process. So, other than on your Low-Carb Days, enjoy them to the fullest.

Your Most Pressing Carb Questions Answered

I spend a lot of my time answering people's questions on various fitness and nutrition topics. I receive countless questions about carbs, and I think the answers to them might serve you as well. So I've included the most common ones here.

Why are carbs good for you?

Carbs are good for you because they play an important role in energy production and help maintain proper thyroid function. When carb consumption is dramatically reduced over several days, thyroid function and thyroid hormones plummet. As a by-product, your metabolism slows down and you feel lethargic and have trouble keeping off the weight.

What good carbs can a diabetic eat?

Any complex carbs rich in fiber and low on the glycemic index will be great for diabetics. Apples, pears, berries, and pretty much all vegetables are great. Legumes such as lentils, beans, and chickpeas are terrific as well. Nonglutinous grains like quinoa can be good substitutes for traditional grains.

What are good carbs for losing weight?

Pretty much the same complex carbs listed above for diabetics to eat. Any carbs that don't spike your blood sugar will be helpful for weight loss.

What are good carbs to eat when working out?

In general, the bulk of your carb consumption should really come after your workout. That's when your muscles are most receptive to the uptake of glucose (the primary building block of carbohydrates). Thus, right after an intense workout is the only time you may want to consider having higher-glycemic carbs like dates, grapes, or even fruit juice. These will help refuel your muscles' and liver's stores of glycogen (stored carbohydrates) and improve your recovery. Additionally, any of the complex carbs that I mentioned above will be good in your overall diet.

How many good carbs should I eat per day?

This is an interesting question, and it really depends on how active you are. As you know, I'm not a fan of counting calories or fussing about grams; however, I'll give you two tips. On a Low-Carb Day (which you can use strategically once per week), I would recommend keeping your net carbs (total carbs minus the fiber) below 50 grams. This will prompt your body to rely more on fat for fuel. On Regular-Cal Days, where carb intake is more liberal, anywhere from 100 to 250 grams is suitable for most people. If you're extremely active (I'm talking intense workouts 5 to 7 days per week), you can get away with 400 to 600 grams of carbs per day.

Fibrous Veggies

Our final category of foods is fibrous veggies. You can literally eat as many of these vegetables as you want. They are very nutrient dense and low in calories, which makes them perfect weight-loss and health-boosting foods, especially for your Low-Cal Days.

This chart shows you which ones to enjoy. It's likely that other suitable (but more rare) vegetables could be included in this chart; however, these are the most common, easily available ones. Note: There really aren't any fibrous veggies to avoid, since this food group is nothing but healthy. As always, do your best to buy organic when possible.

FIBROUS VEGGIES (ENJOY THESE)	
Arugula	Green beans
Bell peppers	Kale
Broccoli	Lettuce and salad greens
Brussels sprouts	
Cabbage	Mushrooms
Cauliflower	Spinach
Celery	Sprouts (bean, broccoli, etc.)
Collard greens	Swiss chard
Cucumber	Zucchini
Eggplant	

Eight or More per Day Keeps the Doctor Away

Did you know that the higher your average daily intake of fruits and vegetables, the lower your chances of developing cardiovascular disease? The largest study of its kind looking at 110,000 men and women revealed that, compared with those in the lowest category of fruit and vegetable intake (less than 1.5 servings a day), those who averaged 8 or more servings a day were 30 percent less likely to have had a heart attack or stroke. The study also found that the most important contributors were leafy green vegetables such as lettuce, spinach, and Swiss chard; cruciferous vegetables such as broccoli, cauliflower, cabbage, Brussels sprouts, bok choy, and kale; and citrus fruits such as oranges, lemons, limes, and grapefruits (and their juices).[14]

Are Raw Cruciferous Veggies Dangerous for Your Thyroid?

Many people reading this book likely suffer from hypothyroidism (underactive thyroid gland). Some might not even be aware of it. We're in the game of burning fat in a healthy way, and how well your thyroid is working is going to have a major impact on your ability to lose weight. After all, your thyroid is your body's master metabolism gland. If it's slow and sluggish, you will be too. And the cells in your body will produce energy (and heat) at a reduced rate, which means you won't be burning as many calories. Thus, a slow thyroid means difficulty with losing weight.

I've often been asked whether raw cruciferous vegetables—kale, broccoli, etc.—negatively impact your thyroid. There's been a lot of debate about this, and I want to give you my opinion, along with some solid science, to provide some important perspective on this topic. However, before I break this down, let me be really straightforward: Very little research supports being scared to eat raw cruciferous vegetables. The popularity of this myth really bothers me, because many of these demonized vegetables have been proven in countless studies to reduce disease. The idea that eating them could be harmful is preposterous. In fact, not eating them will hurt you more.

This myth, though very misguided, did not arise out of thin air. The reason many people are afraid of raw cruciferous veggies has to do with substances called goitrogens, which are mostly present in certain vegetables in their raw state. A goitrogen is a substance that may suppress the function of the thyroid gland by inhibiting iodine uptake in thyroid tissue. Iodine is of crucial importance for the production of thyroid hormone, so naturally anything that suppresses it would be a big concern—if iodine uptake were truly compromised.

Some foods have been shown to be goitrogenic when you eat them in excess or if your iodine intake is low. These mostly include cruciferous vegetables like cabbage, broccoli, Brussels sprouts, cauliflower, bok choy, kale, and collard greens. The thing is, at relatively low concentrations, goitrogens don't have any noticeable impact at all. If you're eating these foods a few times a week, you have absolutely nothing to worry about. However, some experts believe if you start eating them more regularly and you eat them raw (for instance, in a green

Kale for a Clean, Toxin-Clearing Liver

Kale has well-documented cancer- and cardiovascular-protective properties, but did you know that it also plays a significant role in supporting your body's detoxification process? Most toxins that pose a risk to our body must be detoxified by our liver cells using a two-step process. The two steps in the process are called Phase I detoxification and Phase II detoxification. The isothiocyanates made from kale's glucosinolates have been shown to favorably modify both detox steps (Phase I and Phase II).[15] In addition, the unusually large numbers of sulfur compounds in kale have been shown to help support aspects of Phase II detoxification that require the presence of sulfur. By supporting both phases of our cellular detox process, nutrients in kale can give your body an advantage when dealing with toxin exposure, which we know is a potent fat trigger.

smoothie or green juice), goitrogens can actually suppress your thyroid function by inhibiting iodine uptake. Even if this were true—and no human studies have shown it to be true—this suppression can typically be offset by supplementing with iodine and selenium or just eating more iodine-rich foods like sea vegetables.

The reason this whole debate came about in the first place was because a few rodent studies done years ago showed hypothetical thyroid issues from eating very large amounts of cruciferous vegetables. However, it's very important to point out one basic fact: No human study has demonstrated a deficiency in thyroid function from consuming cruciferous vegetables. Only one such study seems to have even been conducted. It found no effects on thyroid function after subjects ate 150 grams of cooked Brussels sprouts daily for 4 weeks—far more than any normal human being would regularly eat!

One case report suggests it would be almost impossible to consume enough cruciferous vegetables to harm the thyroid. In that case, an 88-year-old woman developed hypothyroidism after eating 1 to 1.5 kilograms (2.2 to 3.3 pounds) of raw bok choy every day for several months, which is obviously an excessive and unreasonable intake. The reality is that you would have to consume an insane amount of raw cruciferous vegetables for them to have a negative effect on your thyroid function.

If that doesn't convince you, consider this: Recent results from the Adventist Health Study revealed that vegan Adventists—who consume far more vegetables than the average person and are some of the longest-living people on the planet— were less likely than omnivore Adventists to have hypothyroidism. If plant foods were such a problem, you would think the opposite would be true, right?

As if *that's* not enough, a 2011 study in the *Journal of Clinical Endocrinology and Metabolism* showed that vegans had higher urinary thiocyanate (indicative of higher cruciferous intake) and lower iodine intake, but no difference in thyroid function, which was within the normal range.

If anything, the science proves the opposite of this troublesome myth. Unless you're eating an ungodly amount of raw cruciferous veggies every day, you really have nothing to worry about.

I'm not explaining all of this to push you to eat more raw cruciferous veggies. I am a big advocate of them, but my biggest concern is always that everyone needs to eat more vegetables in general. So if you're still skeptical, then simply steam your greens and raw cruciferous veggies before eating them. Doing so greatly reduces their goitrogenic properties.

In fact, the only cruciferous veggies I eat raw are the ones I put in my morning smoothie or green juice—i.e., kale and other leafy greens. I personally prefer to steam my cruciferous veggies, like broccoli and Brussels sprouts—both of which I love—because in their raw form they're too tough to enjoyably chew!

And here's something else that's very important to keep in mind: Considering that one in two men and one in three women will develop cancer at some point in their lives, it would be crazy not to eat cruciferous vegetables. That's because cruciferous vegetables have been proven to be particularly good at helping fight cancer. Cruciferous vegetables contain glucosinolates and an enzyme called myrosinase. When we blend, chop, or chew these vegetables, we break up the plant cells, allowing myrosinase to come into contact with glucosinolates. This initiates a chemical reaction that produces isothiocyanates (ITCs), powerful anti-cancer compounds.

These ITCs have been shown to detoxify and remove carcinogens, kill cancer cells, and prevent tumors from growing. As I mentioned before, numerous studies have shown that eating cruciferous vegetables protects against all types of cancer. Here are a few examples.

- Twenty-eight servings of vegetables per week (four per day) decreased prostate cancer risk by 33 percent, but just three servings of cruciferous vegetables per week decreased prostate cancer risk by 41 percent.[16]
- One or more servings of cabbage per week decreased the risk of pancreatic cancer by 38 percent.[17]
- One serving per day of cruciferous vegetables reduced the risk of breast cancer by more than 50 percent.[18]

I hope this helps you understand the importance of eating more of these amazingly powerful foods. They're really nothing to be afraid of. If you want something to blame for runaway thyroid problems, then look no further than gluten. This damaging protein found in many grains is strongly correlated with the development of Hashimoto's disease (autoimmune hypothyroidism), which accounts for 90 percent of all cases of hypothyroidism. So don't blame the veggies. They're here to help you. Gluten, on the other hand, really has no redeeming qualities. In no way does it even remotely improve your health. It only harms it.

Now you know the truth about raw cruciferous vegetables, goitrogens, and thyroid function. With this newfound knowledge and reassurance, I'm hoping you can sleep better tonight. Better yet, enjoy the recipes in this book without worrying that eating these health-promoting veggies will do anything but good for your body.

Seven Metabolism-Boosting Foods

If you suspect a sluggish metabolism is the cause of your inability to lose weight, there's a good chance you're right. If you read *The All-Day Fat-Burning Diet*, then you know that what you eat can have a profound impact on your metabolism—good and bad. Keeping your thyroid healthy and building and preserving your muscles are the most important things you can do to ensure a healthy metabolism for as long as possible. However, there are some foods that can help as well. Some of these help your metabolism indirectly by lowering inflammation, while others have a more direct impact by increasing what's called *thermogenesis* (or the production of heat), which directly contributes to burning more fat. What follows is a list of many of the foods you'll be enjoying in this cookbook and how they benefit your metabolism and ability to lose weight.

Ginger

Ginger is one of my very favorite foods. I use it in so many different things I prepare at home, from smoothies to stir-fries. Not only is it an anti-inflammatory spice full of antioxidant properties, it's also one of the most amazing metabolism-boosting foods there is. Its metabolism-boosting traits are due to the unique compounds it contains, most notably gingerol. Gingerol not only aids in digestion but

Ginger Cools Inflammation and Improves Blood Sugar Levels and Exercise Recovery

With inflammation being such a prominent fat trigger (and at the root of many disease processes), any food that can help cool it should be a regular feature in your diet. Ginger is one of the most powerful. A study published in the *Journal of Alternative and Complementary Medicine* revealed that ginger suppresses the pro-inflammatory compounds (cytokines and chemokines) throughout the body.

In a recent study of type 2 diabetics, 2 grams of ginger powder per day lowered fasting blood sugar by 12 percent. It also dramatically improved A1C (a marker for long-term blood sugar levels), leading to a 10 percent reduction over a period of 12 weeks.[19] Ginger's anti-inflammatory benefits have also proven helpful in reducing muscle pain following a workout session. In one study, consuming 2 grams of ginger per day, for 11 days, significantly reduced muscle pain after exercise.[20]

increases body temperature and metabolic rates as much as 20 percent after eating.

Cayenne Pepper

Cayenne is practically bursting with a compound called capsaicin. It will supercharge your metabolism. Capsaicin mildly increases your body temperature, thereby increasing your metabolism and burning fats in the process. Capsaicin also releases endorphins from the brain. These morphinelike molecules naturally occur in the body and create a major feel-good factor once they're released from the brain.

Not only is cayenne one of the best metabolism-boosting foods you can keep around, it also reduces the LDL (bad cholesterol) levels in your blood, thereby lessening your chances of cardiovascular problems. Although cayenne pepper isn't used in any of the recipes in this book, I would encourage you to add some to your evening or morning tea (lemon tea with apple cider vinegar and cayenne is my favorite) or add a little dash to some of the soup recipes if you enjoy the heat.

Cinnamon

Cinnamon isn't just a great topping for apple pie or hot chocolate. It's also an amazing metabolism-boosting food. It contains a generous amount of coumarin, a substance that regulates carbohydrate metabolism in the body. Coumarin also enhances the effects of insulin, thereby increasing the glucose uptake by the tissues in your body. And cinnamon helps in thinning the blood by decreasing its coagulation profile. Those properties alone make cinnamon one of the best metabolism-boosting foods there is, but there's still more: It's also a well-known appetite suppressant, which makes it a tremendous help when it comes to weight management. You'll find cinnamon in many of the recipes throughout this book. It's not only amazing for your health and fat-loss efforts but adds such a wonderful flavor to so many different dishes.

Turmeric

In certain systems of medicine like Ayurveda, turmeric is considered a wonder food, thanks to its abundant anti-inflammatory, antibiotic, and antipyretic properties. A very flavorful spice, turmeric is one of the main ingredients in traditional Indian curry recipes. It is rich in curcumin, which is the most potent inflammation-fighting compound in our food supply. Since inflammation is a big health problem and part of the reason why so many cannot lose weight, reducing inflammation inside your body is a big deal. That's why you'll find this spice in many of the dishes in this cookbook.

Cruciferous Vegetables

Although most of the research on cruciferous vegetables like kale, cauliflower, cabbage, Brussels sprouts, and broccoli tends to highlight their amazing cancer-fighting properties, they also indirectly help you keep the weight off. First, these fibrous veggies are loaded with fiber, which keeps you full longer and prevents you from overeating. Second, they contain sulforaphanes (and other similar compounds) that are vital for your body's detoxification process. This is important because if your body cannot detoxify properly, it will have trouble regulating energy metabolism and blood sugar and removing toxins and excess hormones that build up within it. This toxicity issue is one of the six fat triggers I discussed in *The All-Day Fat-Burning Diet* and is very important. That's why cruciferous vegetables play such a prominent role in these fat-burning recipes.

Coconut Oil

Coconut oil has some unique metabolism-revving properties. That's because it's predominantly made up of medium-chain triglycerides (MCTs), whereas other oils are rich in long-chain triglycerides (LCTs), which are more readily stored than burned. The medium-chain fatty acids have a different metabolic pathway compared to the long-chain fats. Basically, MCTs are more rapidly absorbed by the body and more quickly metabolized (burned) as fuel. The result of this

49 Easy Ways to Eat More Kale

We know that kale is good for us. But just steaming it can get pretty boring, right? So to give you some clever ways to add kale as a side to any of your main dishes, here are 49 easy ways to whip up a yummy kale salad. They're perfect for lunch, potlucks, a dinnertime side, or even dinner itself (just be sure you toss in a handful of nuts to keep your protein intake up!). You'll have dozens of flavor combinations to keep you happy and ensure you're getting plenty of kale. Using this simple table, you can mix and match 49 all-new kale salads! Just take 3 cups of chopped kale or baby kale leaves and add:

1. Your choice of topping combo

2. Your choice of dressing

CHOOSE A KALE TOPPING COMBO	AND ONE DRESSING (add sea salt and pepper to taste, for each)
Cherry tomatoes + diced red onion + kalamata olives	1 tablespoon balsamic vinegar + ½ teaspoon Dijon mustard + 2 tablespoons olive oil
Chopped apples + diced red onion + chopped walnuts + diced celery	2 tablespoons crushed raspberries + 2 tablespoons olive oil + 1 tablespoon apple cider vinegar + 1 tablespoon sesame seeds
Chopped boiled egg + chopped bacon + cherry tomatoes + scallions	2 tablespoons tahini + 1 teaspoon coconut aminos + 1 teaspoon honey
Strawberries + chopped walnuts + diced yellow bell peppers	2 tablespoons lime juice + 1 tablespoon honey + 1 tablespoon coconut cream
Orange and yellow bell peppers + chopped bacon + sliced cucumber	1 tablespoon balsamic vinegar + 1 teaspoon coriander + 1 teaspoon sesame seeds + 1 teaspoon lemon juice + 2 tablespoons olive oil
Brown rice + cannellini beans (rinsed) + chopped red onion	2 tablespoons olive oil + 1 tablespoon lemon juice + 1 clove garlic, crushed and minced
Blueberries + walnuts + sesame seeds	1 tablespoon apple cider vinegar + ½ teaspoon Dijon mustard + 1 tablespoon honey + 2 tablespoons olive oil

Coconut Oil Boosts Your Metabolism

Is it possible that a fat can actually increase your metabolism and help you burn *more* fat? Enter coconut oil, which is chock-full of medium-chain triglycerides (MCTs), shown to provide a major boost to your metabolism. One study found that men who consumed between 1 and 2 tablespoons of coconut oil per day increased their 24-hour energy expenditure by 5 percent.[21] That translates into greater fat burning over time, also corresponding with weight loss. Similar results have been shown in women, with total energy expenditure (i.e., metabolism) increasing after 7 days of a diet composed of 40 percent fat intake (80 percent of which was from MCTs).[22]

accelerated metabolic conversion is that instead of being stored as fat, the calories contained in MCTs are very efficiently converted into fuel for immediate use by your organs and muscles.

Interestingly, MCTs have a slightly lower caloric content than long-chain fats (8.3 calories per gram versus 9 calories per gram, respectively).[23] In addition to their lower caloric content, MCTs are not stored in fat deposits in the body as much as LCTs. Furthermore, MCTs have been shown to enhance thermogenesis (fat burning).[24] So coconut oil and its MCTs seem to offer a triple approach to weight loss: (1) They have a lower calorie content than other fats; (2) they are less likely to be stored as fat; and (3) they contribute to an enhanced metabolism, which burns even more calories.

Hopefully that puts any worries you have about eating more good fat to rest. After all, you'll be seeing a lot of coconut oil throughout this cookbook, and now you know why.

Protein

Okay, this is more of a food *group* than an actual food, but protein's role in helping you lose weight and keeping your metabolic rate up cannot be overlooked.

It's the most important food group you need to know about for this purpose. When it comes to losing weight, curbing cravings, and preserving precious muscle mass, there's one consistent finding in the literature: Protein intake is crucial.

A review article published in 2013 from the Department of Medicine at the Karolinska Institutet in Stockholm, Sweden, looked at 20 weight-loss strategies (drugs, exercise, low-calorie diets, etc.) among overweight and obese individuals. The findings revealed that those subjects who were able to successfully maintain weight loss consumed more protein and even used meal replacement shakes.[25]

Now, unlike most fitness magazines and supplement companies looking to push more of their protein, I'm not going to tell you that you need an obscene amount of protein on a daily basis. The literature indicates that 0.8 to 1.0 gram of protein per kilogram of body weight is more than enough for great health and a lean body (sure, athletes might need a little more). So if you weigh 160 pounds (or 73 kilograms), you would want to average about 58 to 73 grams of protein per day. However, most protein pushers will suggest two to three times that amount, which is absolutely crazy!

For lasting leanness, starting your day with 20 to 30 grams of protein is one of the simplest and most important things you can do, and that's why many of the breakfast and smoothie recipes in this book incorporate a variety of protein sources. Why? Because protein keeps you full longer, which decreases cravings and your desire to eat. Plus it increases your metabolic rate (far more than carbs or fat), which helps you burn more calories.

Research presented at the Obesity Society's annual scientific meeting on November 13, 2013, found that "eating a breakfast rich in protein significantly improves appetite control and may help women to avoid overeating later in the day." The women in this study, aged 18 to 55, consumed either a protein-rich breakfast (with 30 to 39 grams of protein) or a low-protein breakfast (pancakes and syrup) and were then asked to consume a standard lunch meal (whenever they were hungry), eating until they were comfortably full. All breakfast meals contained approximately 300 calories and similar quantities of fat and fiber.

Results of the study showed that participants had improved appetite ratings (lower hunger, more fullness, less desire to eat) throughout the morning and also consumed fewer calories at lunch after eating the protein-rich breakfast rather than the low-protein breakfast.[26] This finding isn't surprising. What does it mean? Starting your day with protein is absolutely crucial for maintaining a healthy, lean body. Throughout this cookbook you'll find various ways to meet your protein requirements, including meats, fish, legumes, nuts, hemp seeds, and even protein powder as an option for some smoothies.

As important as protein is, it's also important not to obsess about it. If, for whatever reason, you don't get enough protein on a particular day, don't worry—you'll be fine. In fact, your liver and muscles have amino acid pools from which they can create complete proteins in times of need or when protein intake is a little lower. What matters most is that your *average* protein intake over time is adequate: not too much, not too little. My promise to you is that as long as you're eating a well-balanced diet including many of the meals in this cookbook, you'll be getting all the protein you need without counting calories or fussing about the little details.

Five Friendly Food Reminders

Now that you have more food knowledge than most doctors and know what basic kitchen staples you'll need, let me give you five friendly food reminders that you should keep in mind as you sift through and try the recipes in this book.

These reminders will serve as your foundation when buying many of the ingredients in the recipes in this book. I'm explaining them here so I don't have to repeat their importance in every single recipe. For instance, ingredients will be listed as "1 cup kale" instead of "1 cup organic kale" or "olive oil" instead of "extra virgin olive oil." Always remember to choose the highest quality of these ingredients whenever possible.

1. Eat Organic Whenever Possible

It should go without saying that to reduce inflammation and toxicity in your body, you should reduce your exposure to pesticides. Thus, do your best to choose organic ingredients whenever possible. If you have the budget to do so, that's great. If not, at least buy the following produce organic if you can, since you'll usually be eating the entire food (skin and all), and thus pesticide residues can't simply be peeled away.

Apples	Hot peppers
Bell peppers	Kale
Blueberries	Lettuce
Celery	Nectarines
Cherries	Peaches
Collard greens	Potatoes
Corn (potential GMO)	Spinach
Cucumbers	Strawberries
Grapes	Yellow squash (potential GMO)
Green beans	Zucchini (potential GMO)
Hawaiian papaya (potential GMO)	

If you're eating produce like bananas and avocados, for instance, where the skin is removed, then buying organic is a little less important. When it comes to animal products (should you choose to eat them), you want to choose what I call "clean proteins." These are meats and eggs that are labeled "wild," "grass fed," "pasture raised," "free range," or "organic." For instance, if you eat salmon, choose wild, not farmed. When choosing beef, go with grass-fed instead of commercially raised. If choosing eggs, go with those from free-range and organically fed chickens instead of chickens that have been cooped up and fed corn. Remember, you are what you eat, so if you're eating animal products, what those animals have been fed truly matters.

→ **Did You Know?** *Red grapes (and red wine) are famous for their antioxidant resveratrol. But they only produce it in response to a fungal infection during their growth. So organic grapes have more resveratrol because they're forced to protect themselves in the absence of pesticide chemicals. Unlike other antioxidants, such as anthocyanins, which give blueberries their color and are an integral part of the fruit, plants produce resveratrol only in response to fungal or bacterial attack. Resveratrol is a natural antibiotic and fungicide, which means that the more natural fungi and bacteria a plant is exposed to, the more resveratrol it will produce. However, if a grape plant is repeatedly sprayed with synthetic fungicides—and grapes are among the most pesticide-intensive crops cultivated—the resveratrol content will be lower. Need another reason to buy organic grapes?*

2. Use BPA-Free Canned Foods

In many of the recipes in this book, you'll see ingredients like beans, legumes, and even full-fat coconut milk that come in a can. For these foods, it's important to choose brands that are organic and use BPA-free cans. In case you didn't know, BPA (bisphenol A) is a toxin that often leaches into drinks and foods sold in bottles and metallic cans. It is a known endocrine disruptor, specifically interfering with the proper functioning of the thyroid. So if you want to keep your metabolism happy, go BPA-free.

3. Use Virgin and Extra Virgin, Cold-Pressed Oils (Organic if Possible)

Many of the recipes call for olive oil or coconut oil. Here again, you want the purest form of these oils. Since coconut oil is much more stable at higher heats, I recommend using it (or butter) for cooking and relying on olive oil for very low-heat cooking or as the main oil in your dressings. When selecting an olive oil, it's important to understand that you're dealing with a monounsaturated fat that can be damaged by excessive light, heat, or oxygen. Thus, the quality and processing of the oil are important to ensure you're not consuming a rancid oil that will do more harm than good inside your body.

Extra virgin olive oil is an unrefined oil and the highest-quality olive oil you can buy. There are very specific standards oil has to meet to receive the "extra virgin" label. Because of the way extra virgin olive oil is made, it retains more true olive taste and contains more of the natural vitamins and minerals found in olives. Extra virgin olive oil is considered an unrefined oil, since it's not treated with chemicals or altered by temperature. The best kinds are cold-pressed. These olive oils typically have a golden-green color, with a distinct flavor and a light peppery finish.

When it comes to coconut oil, there are two main varieties: refined and unrefined. Refined oils are cheaper and possess no coconut flavor or aroma. They are produced from dried copra, not fresh coconuts, and the oil typically undergoes various levels of processing, including being deodorized and bleached. Not good! Unrefined coconut oil is what you want. You'll normally see it labeled as "virgin" (it was incorrectly labeled "extra virgin" in the past), and it possesses a light coconut taste and aroma. Virgin oil is typically made from fresh coconuts and, ideally, made by cold-pressing. Therefore, to benefit from the most value, choose a coconut oil that is virgin (unrefined). I personally use Nutiva's organic virgin coconut oil. As always, for both olive oil and coconut oil, organic is best if you have the option.

4. Drink Unsweetened Almond Milk

There are many brands of almond milk on the market. If you're choosing among them, be sure to pick the unsweetened and unflavored version, since many of the "original" ones contain needless sugar. I like Almond Breeze's almond milk and use it at home if I haven't been able to make any almond milk from scratch (I'll show you how on the next page).

Many people get fussy about premade almond milks because they contain carrageenan, a thickening agent that has been demonized for being a potential carcinogen in rodents, although the research is very sketchy. Some people may react to carrageenan with symptoms like digestive troubles or skin rashes. I find it amusing when people fuss about ingredients like this as they inhale their venti mocha latte or deli sandwich loaded with nitrate-infused meats and gluten-infused bread. We humans are funny creatures with tons of double standards. We are irrational, but you've got to love it. Anyway, as with anything, you're best off making things from scratch. So here's the almond milk recipe that I use at home.

Homemade Almond Milk

Makes 4 cups

1 cup raw almonds
4 cups filtered water
1 pitted Medjool date (optional)
1 teaspoon vanilla extract
Small pinch of sea salt

---

1. Place the almonds in a bowl, cover them with water, and soak them overnight.

2. Rinse and drain the almonds and place them in a blender. Add the filtered water, date (if using), vanilla, and sea salt. Blend at high speed for about 1 minute.

3. Place a nut milk bag over a large bowl and slowly pour the almond milk mixture into the bag. Gently squeeze the bottom of the bag to release the milk. Discard the solids.

4. Pour the filtered almond milk into a glass jar to store in the fridge for 3 to 5 days. Shake the jar very well before using, as the mixture separates when sitting.

Whipped Coconut Cream
and Berries (page 86)

Prosciutto-Wrapped Asparagus
with Fried Eggs (page 93)

Homemade Chocolate Granola
(page 95)

Herbed Smoked Salmon
and Potato Hash (page 118)

Mushroom and Goat Cheese Omelet
(page 92)

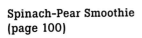

Spinach-Pear Smoothie
(page 100)

Citrus Refresher
(page 110)

Rainbow Sunrise Smoothie
(page 108)

Apple-Kale Salad with
Poppy Seed Dressing (page 138)

Tasty Thai Salad (page 142)

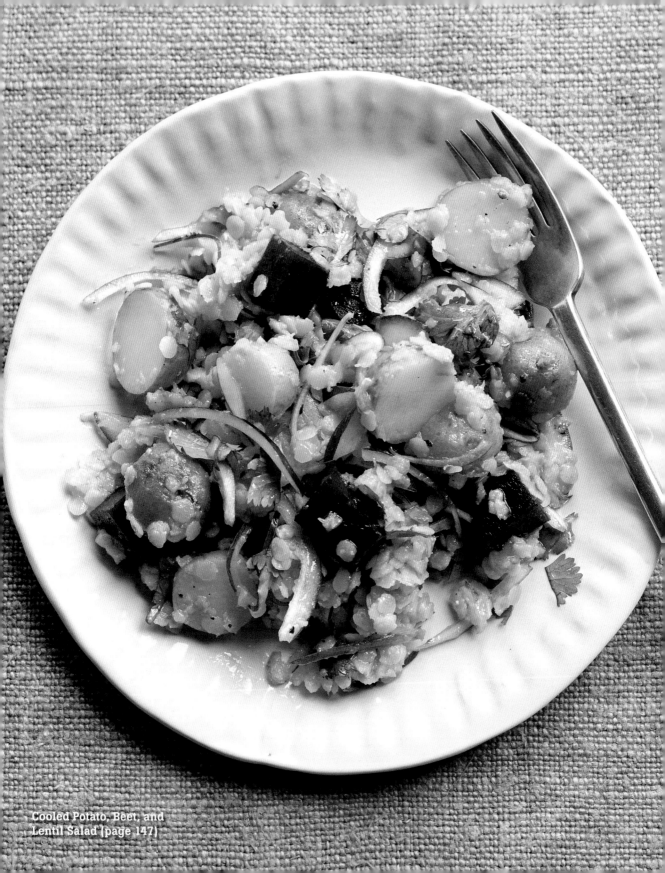

Cooled Potato, Beet, and
Lentil Salad (page 147)

**Citrus and Avocado Salad
(page 151)**

Swiss Chard, Bean, and
Bacon Tahini Salad (page 148)

Vermicelli Garden Bowl
(page 156)

Rainbow Rice Bowl
(page 157)

Flavorful Moroccan Chickpea Soup
(page 173)

Sausage, Tomato, and Kale Soup
(page 176)

No-Cook Ginger Thai Soup
(page 177)

Spicy Black Bean Soup
(page 180)

5. Buy Organic Dried Fruit

Certain recipes in this book call for dried fruit. Since most dried fruits are preserved by the addition of sulfites—an allergen for many people—I recommend using only organic dried fruits, since they do not contain sulfites. A simple way to tell whether dried fruits are organic is to look at their color. For example, dried apricots should turn brown. However, since food manufacturers feel that consumers might react adversely to this color, they use sulfites to retain the apricot's natural orange color. By contrast, organic dried apricots will be brown, and that's what you want.

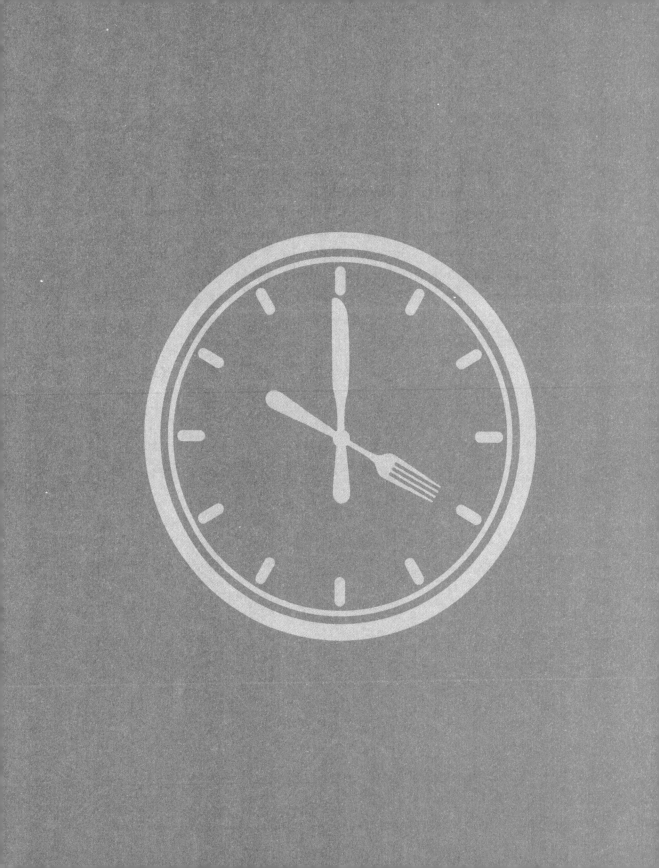

Chapter 4

Breakfasts

FOR SOME, breakfast is the most important meal of the day. But what exactly *is* breakfast? It's the first meal of the day, of course, when you break your fast from the night before. But does that have to be right when you get out of bed, or can you wait several hours before eating? The answer is to listen to your body. If you're hungry, have something to eat (unless it's your 1-Day Fast). If you're not hungry, then wait until you are. It's really that simple. Keep in mind that what you eat for breakfast sets up your day. Foods with poor nutritional value and lots of sugar set you up for feeling drowsy and out of sorts. On the other hand, a healthy breakfast can fuel you for the day ahead by boosting your metabolism, filling you with energy, and kicking any harmful cravings to the curb.

In this chapter, I'm going to hook you up with a dozen of my best breakfast recipes. Most of them provide a good deal of protein, which you want to start your day. Others that incorporate some carbs are well balanced, with protein, fiber, and healthy fats so your blood sugar doesn't go crazy. And a few others are nice treats, especially on your feast days.

Are you ready to start your day on the right foot? Let's go!

Whipped Coconut Cream and Berries

Makes 2 servings

1 can (14 ounces) organic
full-fat coconut milk,
chilled

2 tablespoons xylitol or
erythritol (optional)

1 tablespoon ground
cinnamon

1 tablespoon vanilla
extract

2 cups berries of your
choice

I love tricking my kids (when it's good for them). And this
is one dessertlike breakfast that gets them every time.
They think they're having a dessert, when in reality
they're enjoying a rich breakfast full of healthy fats and
tons of antioxidants. It's a great alternative to yogurt.
You can even enjoy this as an after-dinner treat. For best
results, keep the can of coconut milk in the fridge for
several hours ahead of time.

1. Into a medium bowl, scoop the coconut milk solids (the
   thick, creamy part). Discard the liquid. Add the xylitol or
   erythritol (if using), cinnamon, and vanilla.

2. Beat the coconut milk mixture with an electric mixer for
   2 minutes, or until peaks form and the desired whipped
   cream consistency is achieved.

3. Pour the berries into a separate bowl, top with the whipped
   cream, and enjoy!

Coconut–Mango Chia Seed Pudding

Makes 4 servings

2 cups unsweetened almond milk

½ cup chia seeds

1 teaspoon vanilla extract

⅓ cup unsweetened shredded coconut

1 mango, diced

Chia seeds absorb liquid like nobody's business, which is part of the reason why they're such a good source of fiber, great for absorbing toxins from your digestive tract and removing them from your body. Plus, they're a great source of omega-3 fatty acids. The easiest way to eat more chia seeds is in pudding form—like this recipe. Here, the combination of coconut and mango makes this high-fiber breakfast a tasty treat. It is best prepared the night before so that it's ready to go first thing in the morning.

1. In a jar or container with a lid, place the almond milk, chia seeds, vanilla, and coconut. Cover and shake well to combine ingredients. Refrigerate overnight (or for at least 4 hours).

2. When ready to serve, scoop the now-thickened chia seed pudding into a bowl, top with the mango, and enjoy.

Apple-Cinnamon Chia Seed Pudding

Makes 4 servings

½ cup chia seeds

2 cups full-fat canned
coconut milk

1 tablespoon vanilla
extract

Pinch of sea salt

1 tablespoon coconut oil

1 medium apple, sliced

1 teaspoon ground
cinnamon

¼ cup raisins

¼ cup chopped almonds

2 tablespoons hemp seeds

¼ cup shredded coconut

If you're more of an apple and cinnamon type of person, then you'll love this chia seed pudding. It's a great substitute for the traditional apple and cinnamon oatmeal that many people turn to for breakfast. This recipe keeps things relatively low carb and high fiber and healthy fat, which will fuel you for hours without raising fat-storing insulin levels (like oatmeal would).

1. In a mason jar, combine the chia seeds, coconut milk, vanilla, and sea salt. Stir, cover, and refrigerate overnight.

2. In a medium skillet over medium heat, melt the coconut oil. Add the apple slices, cinnamon, and a pinch of sea salt. Cook, stirring frequently, until the apples are tender and caramelized, about 10 minutes.

3. Place the chia pudding in a bowl and top with the apples, raisins, almonds, hemp seeds, and coconut. Enjoy!

Fried Egg Breakfast Hash

Makes 4 servings

1 tablespoon butter or
  coconut oil

1 medium sweet potato,
  peeled and cubed

1 medium green bell
  pepper, seeded and
  diced

1 medium onion, sliced

2 cups chopped spinach or
  Swiss chard

4 slices bacon

4 eggs

1 teaspoon sea salt

½ teaspoon ground black
  pepper

If you're tired of the same boring eggs for breakfast, then this hash will be a breath of fresh air. It's super simple to make. Simply sauté your veggies, then top with fried eggs. It's easy and loaded with great nutrition and even better flavors.

1. In a large skillet over medium heat, melt the butter or coconut oil. Add the sweet potato, green pepper, and onion and cook, stirring frequently, until softened, 5 to 7 minutes. Stir in the spinach or Swiss chard and cook for another 2 minutes.

2. Meanwhile, in a separate skillet over medium heat, cook the bacon until lightly crisped, about 4 minutes on each side. Place the bacon in a bowl lined with paper towels. Chop it into 1" pieces.

3. Discard some of the bacon fat from the second skillet, but keep 2 tablespoons. Crack the eggs into the skillet and fry them over medium heat for 3 minutes, or until the whites are set. Sprinkle to taste with salt and pepper.

4. Divide the sautéed veggies and bacon among 4 plates and top with the fried eggs.

The Right Way to Crack an Egg

When you're cracking open your eggs, do so on a flat surface, like the counter, rather than on the rim of a bowl. That's because breaking them on the rim of a bowl causes more shell shatter and can sometimes drive tiny pieces of shell into the egg whites. Cracking your eggs on the counter minimizes this collateral damage.

Hemp Seed Porridge

Makes 2 servings

2 cups almond milk

½ cup hemp seeds

2 tablespoons chia seeds

¼ teaspoon ground cinnamon

2 tablespoons almond butter

¼ cup chopped almonds

1 apple, sliced (not recommended for Low-Carb Days)

I grew up on Cream of Wheat for breakfast. At the time, I didn't understand why my stomach was so gassy and bloated for hours after my bowl of creamy wheat. Now I do. Gluten (which is found in wheat) is bad news, and that's why it's not part of the All-Day Fat-Burning recipe philosophy. Thankfully, this hemp seed porridge is a terrific alternative to that traditional morning staple. Not only is it gluten-free, but it's also loaded with protein and fiber to keep you full for hours and keep those sugar cravings at bay.

1. In a medium saucepan over medium heat, bring the almond milk to a simmer. Stir in the hemp seeds, chia seeds, and cinnamon. Simmer lightly for 5 minutes, stirring occasionally.

2. Turn off the heat and stir in the almond butter. Top with the chopped almonds and apple slices (if using) and serve.

Protein-Packed Morning Muesli with Applesauce

Makes 2 servings

Applesauce

3 apples, peeled and diced

¼ cup water

1 teaspoon ground cinnamon

½ teaspoon ground nutmeg

¼ teaspoon grated fresh ginger

Pinch of salt

Muesli

¼ cup coconut oil

1 cup gluten-free oats

¼ cup chopped almonds

¼ cup chopped walnuts or pecans

2 tablespoons pumpkin seeds

1 tablespoon maple syrup

3 tablespoons hemp seeds

1 tablespoon ground flaxseeds

1 teaspoon ground cinnamon

1 teaspoon ground nutmeg

½ apple, chopped

Want a high-protein breakfast option other than eggs? Try this nut-based muesli on for size. This recipe will give you about 15 grams of vegan-based protein per serving and appease that little sweet tooth, thanks to the easy-to-make applesauce.

1. *To make the applesauce:* In a medium pot over medium-high heat, combine the apples, water, cinnamon, nutmeg, ginger, and salt. Bring to a boil, then reduce the heat and simmer, covered, for about 15 minutes.

2. Remove the pot from the heat. Lightly mash the applesauce or blend it in a blender (depending on the consistency that you want). Keep covered to keep warm.

3. *To make the muesli:* Meanwhile, in a large skillet over medium heat, melt the coconut oil. Add the oats, almonds, walnuts or pecans, and pumpkin seeds. Toast for 10 minutes, or until fragrant and golden, stirring often. Add the maple syrup toward the end of the toasting process. Remove the pan from the heat and stir in the hemp seeds, flaxseeds, cinnamon, nutmeg, and chopped apple.

4. Serve by dividing the muesli between 2 bowls and topping it with the applesauce.

Mushroom and Goat Cheese Omelet

Low Carb, Low Cal

Makes 1 serving

1 tablespoon butter

1 cup chopped cremini or
white button
mushrooms, stemmed

1 clove garlic, minced

1 teaspoon sea salt,
divided

2 large eggs

Ground black pepper

1 teaspoon chopped fresh
tarragon (optional)

1 tablespoon chopped
parsley

1–2 tablespoons goat
cheese

I don't often recommend cheese, but when I do, it's goat cheese, which is much less problematic for our health and waistlines than regular dairy. Plus the goat cheese simply brings this omelet to life. If you don't want to add the cheese, then that's cool as well. Just enjoy the omelet with the mushrooms.

1. In a large skillet over medium heat, melt the butter. Add the mushrooms and cook, stirring frequently, for 5 minutes, or until they're nicely browned and tender, adding more butter if needed. Stir in the garlic and ½ teaspoon of the salt and continue cooking until fragrant, about 1 minute.

2. Meanwhile, in a medium bowl, whisk together the eggs, the remaining ½ teaspoon salt, pepper to taste, and tarragon (if using) until well combined.

3. Pour the eggs on top of the mushrooms and spread them evenly throughout the skillet. Using a spatula, lift the egg mixture around the sides of the skillet to allow more of the egg to fill in underneath.

4. As the eggs begin to solidify, after about 2 minutes, add the parsley and goat cheese. Flip one side of the omelet over the other. Cook for 1 more minute, then serve.

Prosciutto-Wrapped Asparagus with Fried Eggs

Low Carb

Makes 2 servings

½ cup water

8 asparagus shoots, trimmed

1 tablespoon butter

4 eggs

1 teaspoon sea salt

Ground black pepper

4 slices prosciutto

Hold on to your seat, because this breakfast is going to rock your world. In just a few minutes and using just a few ingredients, you'll whip up a meal that will make you feel like a gourmet chef. If you have a special someone you want to impress, then this is the breakfast for him or her. The key to this recipe is getting the asparagus just right. You don't want it either chewy or too tough, so be sure to follow the instructions and check it throughout—it will be well worth it. The prosciutto is a delicious addition that takes a bland-tasting green veggie and brings it to life. If you've got kids, I bet they'll enjoy this too.

1. Pour the water into a large skillet over medium heat. Add the asparagus. Cover, bring to a boil, then reduce to a simmer. Cook the asparagus until tender, about 5 minutes. Drain and set aside.

2. In another large skillet over medium heat, melt the butter. Crack the eggs into the pan, ensuring that the yolks do not break. Sprinkle with the salt and with pepper to taste. Cook for 2 minutes, or until the desired consistency is achieved.

3. Meanwhile, wrap 2 shoots of asparagus in 1 slice of prosciutto. Continue until you have made 4 wraps. Divide them between 2 plates. Once the eggs are ready, place 2 eggs on top of each plate of prosciutto-wrapped asparagus. Serve with a side of mixed greens (if desired), and dig in.

Cherry-Coconut Granola

Makes about 6 cups

¼ cup coconut oil, melted
+ additional to grease
the pan

1 teaspoon vanilla extract

¼ cup honey or maple
syrup

1 cup unsweetened
coconut flakes

½ cup raw sunflower seeds

1 cup chopped almonds

1 cup chopped pecans

1 cup unsweetened dried
cherries

1 teaspoon ground
cinnamon

Sea salt

Most store-bought granola is nothing more than expensive candy with heaps of sugar and other unnecessary ingredients. The good news is that you can make a much healthier granola in minutes that can last for days. In this one, the nuts, seeds, and cinnamon mitigate the sugar from the cherries and honey or maple syrup.

1. Preheat the oven to 350°F and grease a 13" x 9" baking sheet with coconut oil.

2. In a small bowl, whisk the ¼ cup melted coconut oil, vanilla, and honey or maple syrup. In a medium bowl, mix the coconut flakes, sunflower seeds, almonds, pecans, cherries, cinnamon, and salt to taste. Pour the coconut oil mixture over the dry granola ingredients and mix well.

3. Pour the granola onto the baking sheet and bake for 15 to 20 minutes, until the granola is golden brown. Allow the granola to cool and serve it with almond milk or full-fat coconut milk.

Granola Tips

- To ensure even baking, spread the granola evenly on the baking sheet.

- Avoid baking the granola until completely crisp or it will taste burned. It should come out a little soft and will firm up as it cools.

- For added crispness, let the granola cool in the oven with the door ajar.

- Granola can be stored for about 3 weeks in an airtight container.

Homemade Chocolate Granola

Makes about 10 cups

3 tablespoons butter, melted + 1 tablespoon to grease the baking sheets

3 cups gluten-free rolled oats

1 cup chopped almonds

1 cup chopped pecans

½ cup chopped cashews

½ cup chopped hazelnuts

1 tablespoon raw cacao powder

1 teaspoon sea salt

¼ cup honey or maple syrup

1 tablespoon pure vanilla extract

¼ cup raw cacao nibs or unsweetened chocolate chips

Like most kids of my generation, I grew up eating copious amounts of junk. My breakfast cereals were like candy bars floating in milk. No wonder I felt like a zombie half the time. Thankfully, this granola is a healthy breakfast treat that actually does your body good. In fact, it's a staple in my cupboard. It's so darn good and filling, especially when served with full-fat coconut milk. Add some chopped strawberries if you feel like cutting the chocolate taste a little bit. Like the previous granola, this protein-rich granola can be stored in an airtight container for up to 3 weeks.

1. Preheat the oven to 325°F. Use 1 tablespoon of butter to grease 2 large rimmed baking sheets.

2. In a large bowl, mix the oats, almonds, pecans, cashews, hazelnuts, cacao powder, and salt. In a smaller bowl, whisk the melted butter, honey or maple syrup, and vanilla. Pour the butter mixture over the oat mixture and stir with a spoon until well combined.

3. Divide the mixture between the 2 baking sheets, spreading it in an even layer. Bake for 20 minutes, then stir. Bake for another 10 to 15 minutes, or until the oats are golden brown and the nuts look well toasted—don't overcook. Just before the end of the cooking time, stir in the cacao nibs or chocolate chips.

4. Let the granola cool completely in the pans. The oats may feel soft but will crisp up as they cool. Enjoy the granola in a bowl with almond milk or full-fat coconut milk for a filling breakfast that will keep you going for hours.

Yuri's Famous Crepes

Makes 8

1 cup buckwheat flour

½ cup tapioca starch

2 eggs

3 cups almond milk

2 teaspoons vanilla extract

Pinch of sea salt

Hazelnut spread or peanut
butter (optional)

For years, I've wowed friends and family with these gluten-free crepes. Having also lived in France during my soccer years, I can tell you without hesitation that these crepes are even better than the ones you'd find at a creperie in Paris. Seriously! These crepes are dangerously good, so they should ideally be saved for your 1-Day Feast. Yes, they go against my "limit carbs in the morning" recommendation but, as a rare treat, they're okay.

1. Preheat the oven to 250°F. In a large bowl, combine the flour, starch, eggs, almond milk, vanilla, and salt. Mix well to form a runny batter.

2. Place a large skillet over high heat. Add enough butter to grease the skillet. Pour 1 ladleful of batter into the skillet, then move the pan around so that the batter covers its entire surface.

3. Cook the crepe until small bubbles begin to form, about 2 minutes. Then flip it, reduce the heat to medium, and cook for 2 more minutes. If you're adding hazelnut spread or peanut butter, spread it on top of the crepe during the final minute of cooking so that it warms and melts. Yum!

4. Continue making crepes until all the batter has been used. Keep finished crepes warm in the oven. To serve, plate the crepes, add your favorite toppings, roll up, and enjoy.

Soft-Boiled Egg and Avocado Bowl

Makes 1 serving

2 eggs

½ avocado, chopped

1 tablespoon olive oil

2 teaspoons lemon juice

**Salt and ground black
    pepper**

This is a terrific high-protein, high–healthy fat breakfast for busy mornings. It will keep you satisfied for hours and keep away those midmorning carb cravings. Soft-boiled eggs not only take less time to make than fried eggs, but they're easier for your stomach to digest.

1. Fully submerge the eggs in a medium pot of cold water. Then set the pot over medium-high heat until the water starts to simmer. Simmer the eggs for 2 to 4 minutes. Do not let the water boil, since that will crack the eggs. Adjust the heat to maintain a simmer.

2. Remove the pot from the stove top, drain, and run under cold water in the sink for a few minutes until the eggs are barely warm.

3. Peel the eggs, then cut them into quarters and place them in a bowl. Add the chopped avocado. Drizzle with the olive oil, lemon juice, and salt and pepper to taste, and enjoy!

Chapter 5

Smoothies

QUICK, HOW MANY fruits and vegetables did you eat yesterday?

You should be aiming for 8 to 12 servings a day. That's because a healthy body is best fueled by raw, fresh produce. Still, most people struggle to eat even just a few servings of fruits and veggies in a day. Well, smoothies are a fantastic way to boost your fruit and vegetable intake, because it's a lot easier to drink 4 to 6 servings of vegetables and fruit than it is to eat them. The smoothies in this chapter are very well balanced, with healthy carbs (fruit), protein, and fiber. This means that they'll keep you full longer and not spike your blood sugar.

For any of these smoothies, feel free to add additional water (or nut milk) to make them more liquid, if desired. Also, if you have any raw potato starch on hand, you can add 1 tablespoon to any of the smoothies without altering their taste. As mentioned earlier, this form of resistant starch is an easy way to provide the good bacteria in your gut with their preferred source of fuel and improve your overall health in the process.

Spinach-Pear Smoothie

Makes 2 servings

2 cups almond milk

1 pear, cored and
quartered

2 tablespoons hemp seeds

1 tablespoon ground
flaxseeds

1" piece fresh ginger,
peeled and grated, juice
reserved

2 cups baby spinach

What brings this green smoothie to life is the ginger. Not only is ginger an amazing anti-inflammatory food, it also provides a zingy kick to a recipe. This smoothie is a classic example. The hemp seeds provide a good helping of protein, and the ground flaxseeds add some extra fiber to keep you full longer.

In a blender, combine the almond milk, pear, hemp seeds, flaxseeds, grated ginger and reserved juice, and spinach. Blend for 20 seconds, or until smooth.

Cabbage Patch Smoothie

Low Cal

Makes 2 servings

2 cups almond milk

1 cup chopped red cabbage

1½ cups blueberries (fresh or frozen)

2 tablespoons almonds

¼ teaspoon almond extract

½ tablespoon maple syrup

Did you know that cabbage is one of the best food sources of glutamine? The reason that matters to you is because glutamine is the single most important amino acid for repairing the cells in your gut. Plus it's needed for muscle repair. Cabbage has a naturally fiery flavor, but the blueberries and hint of maple syrup in this recipe bring the flavors of the cabbage to life.

In a blender, combine the almond milk, cabbage, blueberries, almonds, almond extract, and maple syrup. Blend for 20 seconds, or until smooth.

Cool Green Smoothie

Makes 2 servings

1 cup pineapple chunks

1 cup honeydew melon chunks

2 cups spinach

2 tablespoons hemp seeds

1 tablespoon ground flaxseeds

1 cup water

1 cup coconut water

¼ cup mint leaves

If you're worried about the sugar from the fruit in this smoothie, don't be. The protein and fiber from the hemp and flax bring things into balance. However, since this is a little high in fruit, I would recommend saving this smoothie for after a workout or using it as a meal or snack option on your 1-Day Feast. You'll love what the coconut water and mint do to this smoothie. So refreshing, especially after a good sweat.

In a blender, combine the pineapple, melon, spinach, hemp seeds, flaxseeds, water, coconut water, and mint leaves. Blend for 20 seconds, or until smooth.

Berry-Peach Smoothie

Makes 2 servings

2 cups almond milk

1 cup water or coconut water

1 cup frozen berries

1 peach, pitted

1 cup packed baby spinach

2 tablespoons hemp seeds

1 tablespoon ground flaxseeds

2 tablespoons cashew butter

1 teaspoon vanilla extract

2 or 3 drops liquid stevia (optional)

I find that peaches seem to be losing favor. Few people eat them nowadays. However, this smoothie will make you fall in love with peaches once again. Together with the berries, the peach perfectly masks the spinach packed within. Thus, this can serve as a great nutrient-rich smoothie for kids who have an aversion to anything green.

In a blender, combine the almond milk, water or coconut water, berries, peach, spinach, hemp seeds, flaxseeds, cashew butter, vanilla, and stevia (if using). Blend for 20 seconds, or until smooth.

Swap Your Soda for This

If you're a self-proclaimed soda lover and want a healthier alternative that is a little more exciting than just water, then try this Apple Cider Vinegar Soda recipe. Mix 2 generous cups of water with 2 tablespoons of apple cider vinegar and the juice of half a lemon. This is a wonderful digestive aid before (or with) a meal and helps to satisfy that "fizzy bubbly" craving.

Fill-Up-the-Tank Smoothie

Makes 2 servings

1 cup almond milk

1 cup full-fat canned
coconut milk

1 cup frozen berries

2 tablespoons hemp seeds

1 tablespoon ground
flaxseeds

1 teaspoon ground
cinnamon

2 or 3 drops liquid stevia
(optional)

Warning: This is a seriously filling smoothie. I would reserve this for a 1-Day Feast or for after an intense workout. On our fat-burning journey, it's important to remember that the occasional calorie-rich meal is not only okay but highly recommended to keep your thyroid and other hormones happy. With that in mind, please enjoy this thick and creamy smoothie without the guilt.

In a blender, combine the almond milk, coconut milk, berries, hemp seeds, flaxseeds, cinnamon, and stevia (if using). Blend for 20 seconds, or until smooth.

Tropical Green Smoothie

Makes 2 servings

1 cup unsweetened
   coconut water

1 cup water

3 cups spinach

1 cup frozen pineapple

½ mango, chopped

½ avocado

2 tablespoons hemp seeds

1" piece fresh ginger,
   peeled and grated, juice
   reserved

I've been to Mexico many times in my life. There's something I just love about the country, the people, and the flavors. That's probably why many of my recipes are inspired by Mexican flavor and ingredient combinations. This smoothie brings together hints of Mexico in a substantial drink that will keep you full for hours. As a result, please reserve this for a breakfast, 1-Day Feast meal, or postworkout snack or meal.

In a blender, combine the coconut water, water, spinach, pineapple, mango, avocado, hemp seeds, and grated ginger and reserved juice. Blend for 20 seconds, or until smooth.

Chocolate Protein Smoothie

Low Carb

Makes 2 to 3 servings

1 can (14 ounces) full-fat
coconut milk

2 cups water

2 handfuls spinach

¼ cup almonds

2 tablespoons hemp seeds

1 tablespoon ground
flaxseeds

1 tablespoon raw cacao
powder

1 scoop protein powder of
your choice (unflavored
or chocolate works
best)

If you like chocolate and want a high-protein smoothie, then this is it. Plus it's low carb, so it's perfect for a Low-Carb Day. As with many of the other smoothies in this book, you're getting a lot of stuff in here: healthy fats, protein, fiber, and great flavor. Because it is quite substantial, I would recommend this as a standalone breakfast on any day or after a workout.

In a blender, combine the coconut milk, water, spinach, almonds, hemp seeds, flaxseeds, cacao powder, and protein powder. Blend for 20 seconds, or until smooth.

Vanilla-Cashew-Ginger Smoothie

Makes 3 servings

1 banana

1 cup cashews

2 scoops vanilla protein
powder

3 cups water

2 tablespoons hemp seeds

1 tablespoon flaxseed oil

1 tablespoon ground
flaxseeds

1 teaspoon ground
cinnamon

2" piece fresh ginger,
peeled

6 ice cubes

This is a dangerously good smoothie. When our kids ask for a treat, we give them this instead. And to be honest, they don't even know the difference. The combination of cashew, vanilla, and ginger is surprisingly awesome. It's a thick and filling smoothie, so it's perfect for those times when you're feeling like something with a little more oomph. And, as with all the other smoothies, it's perfect for after a workout.

In a blender, combine the banana, cashews, protein powder, water, hemp seeds, oil, flaxseeds, cinnamon, ginger, and ice cubes. Blend for 20 seconds, or until smooth.

Bananas That Burn Fat?

Not all bananas are created equal. Remember that unripe bananas are exceptionally high in a very beneficial carbohydrate called resistant starch, which degrades as the banana ripens. Resistant starch is a type of starch that is not digested in the small intestine and passes to the large intestine, where it serves as fuel for your gut bacteria. Research has shown that resistant starch intake decreases blood sugar and insulin after eating, lowers cholesterol and blood triglycerides, makes your cells more sensitive to insulin, increases satiety, and reduces fat storage.[1] Pretty amazing, if you ask me. You can also get resistant starch from cooked, then cooled, potatoes, beans, and rice, as well as by adding 1 to 2 tablespoons of raw potato starch (found in powdered format at a health food store) to water or a smoothie.

Rainbow Sunrise Smoothie

Makes 2 servings

1 cup frozen peaches

1 cup water or coconut
water, divided

1 cup frozen raspberries

1 cup blueberries

1 frozen banana

½ cup almond milk

3 cups spinach and/or
1 scoop Yuri Elkaim's
Energy Greens
(yurigreens.com)

1 tablespoon chia seeds

1 tablespoon ground
flaxseeds

1 tablespoon hemp seeds

4 or 5 drops liquid stevia
(optional)

½ cup diced fresh peaches
and berries

How this smoothie got its name will be revealed if you follow the instructions closely. Sure, you could just whip everything together in the blender, but then you'd miss the "sunrise." The joy of this smoothie comes in the layering (as detailed in the recipe). If you want to impress anyone (including yourself) with a good-looking and great-tasting smoothie, then this is the one.

1. In a blender, puree the frozen peaches and ⅓ cup of the water or coconut water for 20 seconds. Spoon into the bottoms of 2 large glasses.

2. Add the frozen raspberries to the blender, along with another ⅓ cup of the water or coconut water. Puree for 20 seconds. Spoon on top of the peach mixture.

3. Add the blueberries and the remaining ⅓ cup of the water or coconut water to the blender and puree for 20 seconds. Spoon on top of the raspberry mixture. Rinse out the blender.

4. In the clean blender, combine the banana, almond milk, spinach and/or Energy Greens, chia seeds, flaxseeds, hemp seeds, and stevia (if using). Puree for 20 seconds, or until smooth. Spoon on top of the blueberry layer. Add the diced peaches and berries, and enjoy.

Crazy Coconut Smoothie

Low Cal

Makes 2 servings

¼ pineapple

1 handful spinach

3 cups coconut water

2 tablespoons Yuri
   Elkaim's Energy Greens

1 tablespoon ground
   flaxseeds

2 tablespoons hemp seeds

4 or 5 ice cubes

Coconut water is Mother Nature's sports drink. It has almost the same electrolyte balance as the interstitial fluid in our body. For that reason, it's a great beverage to enjoy after a sweat-inducing workout. And if you're not a fan of greens, then coconut water's natural sweet flavor can make them more palatable than plain water or almond milk. This recipe also calls for my Energy Greens. If you don't have them, no big deal—just make the smoothie without them.

In a blender, combine the pineapple, spinach, coconut water, Energy Greens, flaxseeds, hemp seeds, and ice cubes. Blend for 20 seconds, or until smooth.

Citrus Refresher

Makes 2 servings

2 whole unpeeled oranges

1 cup peeled, chopped
    cucumber

2 tablespoons Yuri
    Elkaim's Energy Greens

1" piece fresh ginger,
    peeled and grated

1 tablespoon ground
    flaxseeds

2 tablespoons hemp seeds

2 cups water

4 ice cubes

Cucumber, oranges, ginger. That sounds like a weird combination, doesn't it? However, you might think otherwise after drinking this smoothie. As its name implies, this drink is refreshing and perfect for a warm summer's day. The Energy Greens enhance the flavor, yet the smoothie is terrific even without them.

In a blender, combine the oranges, cucumber, Energy Greens, ginger, flaxseeds, hemp seeds, water, and ice cubes. Blend for 20 seconds, or until smooth.

Vanilla Protein "Milkshake"

Makes 2 servings

2 cups almond milk

1 frozen banana

1 tablespoon peanut butter

2 scoops vanilla protein powder or 2 scoops unflavored protein powder + 1 teaspoon vanilla extract

Back in my university days, I loved going to nightclubs to listen and dance to world-renowned DJs working their magic. We would often leave the club at 2 a.m., naturally famished. In Toronto, there was a restaurant we could always count on to provide an indulgent post-clubbing early morning meal. It was a 24-hour diner that made, among other great items, the best milkshakes in the world. This smoothie was inspired by those late-night milkshake memories, although my version is much, much healthier. Instead of making you feel bloated and packing thousands of calories, this healthier "milkshake" is high in protein and perfect at any point of the day.

In a blender, combine the almond milk, banana, peanut butter, and vanilla protein powder or unflavored protein powder plus vanilla. Blend for 20 seconds, or until smooth.

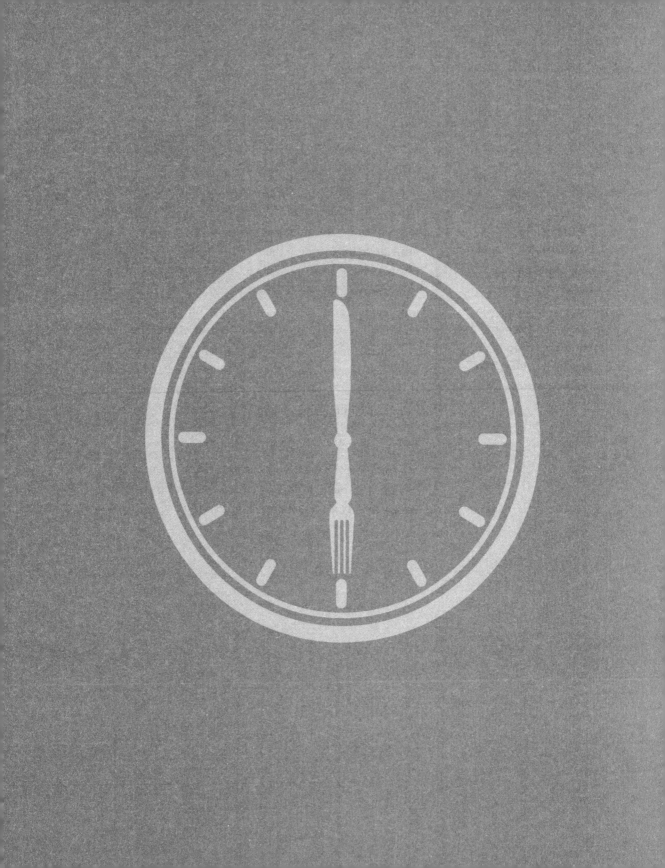

Chapter 6

Sides

SOMETIMES IT'S NICE to have a healthy selection of side dishes to choose from to go alongside your main courses. And many of the sides in this chapter are substantial enough on their own to be a smaller meal (perhaps on a Low-Cal Day). I've got sides to cover all your needs, from rice substitutes to healthy fries to potato salads that actually burn fat, and more.

In general, if your main course doesn't have enough substance for your liking, then pair it with one of these sides to get more of what you need. If a particular main is a little low in veggies, then choose a side (or salad) that will fill that gap so you're eating well-balanced meals as often as possible.

Cauliflower Rice

Makes 8 cups

**1 head cauliflower,
chopped into florets**

2 tablespoons coconut oil

**½ cup vegetable or
chicken broth**

This is a terrific grain-free alternative to rice and perfect for any Low-Carb Day or Low-Cal Day. When we have friends over for lunch or dinner, we'll often make vegan sushi, which uses this Cauliflower Rice instead of traditional rice. When we tell them that the base is cauliflower and not actual rice, they're amazed at how good it is. I think you'll feel the same way too.

1. In a blender or food processor, place a small handful of the cauliflower. Process for 20 seconds, or until the cauliflower is the consistency of rice. Repeat until all of the cauliflower is processed.

2. Place a large skillet over medium heat. Melt the coconut oil. Add the cauliflower rice and broth and cook, covered, for 2 to 3 minutes, or until the cauliflower becomes soft. Turn the heat off, let the cauliflower cool slightly, and serve it with your favorite dish!

Salt and Vinegar Parsnip "Fries"

1 pound parsnips, peeled

2 tablespoons coconut oil, melted

1 teaspoon sea salt

½ teaspoon ground black pepper

1 tablespoon malt vinegar

½ tablespoon liquid honey

½ tablespoon horseradish

½ tablespoon whole grain mustard

Do you like salt and vinegar chips? I do. Sadly, other than tasting good, they do little for us but pack on the pounds. I made it my mission to find a healthier substitute. And that's exactly what I did with these Salt and Vinegar Parsnip "Fries." In case you've never had them, parsnips are related to the mighty carrot, yet their taste is more neutral—perfect for an alternative to potato-based fries or chips. These fries work really well with any red meat dishes, including many of the mains in this cookbook. You can also make a bunch of them and enjoy the leftovers as an on-the-go snack. However, because they are a starchy carb, you'll want to avoid these on your Low-Carb Days. Any other day is fine, however.

1. Preheat the oven to 425°F. Cut the parsnips into ¼" fries. In a large bowl, toss the parsnips with the coconut oil, sea salt, and pepper.

2. On a baking sheet lined with parchment paper, spread the parsnips in a single layer. Bake for 25 to 30 minutes, or until the tips become golden brown.

3. Meanwhile, in a small bowl, stir together the vinegar, honey, horseradish, and mustard. Drizzle the sauce over the hot fries and serve.

Sweet Potato Salad

Makes 4 servings

Dressing

3 tablespoons apple cider
vinegar

1 tablespoon honey

2 teaspoons Dijon mustard

1 teaspoon poppy seeds

½ teaspoon sea salt

½ teaspoon ground black
pepper

2 tablespoons olive oil

¼ cup diced red onion
(about ¼ medium onion)

Salad

1 pound sweet potatoes
(about 2 medium),
peeled

2 tablespoons coconut oil,
melted

1 teaspoon sea salt

½ teaspoon ground black
pepper

1 teaspoon grated fresh
ginger

⅓ cup sliced radishes

⅓ cup chopped pickles

¼ cup chopped scallions

This healthy-carb salad is loaded with an array of odd flavors that come together beautifully. Sweet potatoes are a terrific starchy carb (especially for active individuals) and provide a whopping amount of vitamin A. I find that their natural sweet taste can sometimes be a little much if you're eating them alone. Yet, in this recipe, the addition of ginger, radishes, pickles, scallions, and an amazing dressing turns the boring sweet potato into a rock star. This salad is great on its own or alongside any lighter main course.

1. *To make the dressing:* In a large bowl, whisk together the vinegar, honey, mustard, poppy seeds, salt, and pepper. While whisking constantly, slowly add the oil until all of it is incorporated. Add the onion, stir to combine, and set aside.

2. *To make the salad:* Coat a grill rack or broiler-pan rack with coconut oil. Preheat the grill or broiler. Cut the sweet potatoes widthwise into ¼" slices. In a large bowl, toss the potatoes with the coconut oil, sea salt, and pepper. Grill on greased (with coconut oil) pan or grill, turning once, for 10 to 12 minutes, or until tender.

3. Meanwhile, in a small bowl, stir together the ginger, radishes, pickles, and scallions.

4. Arrange the grilled potatoes on a plate. Top with the radish mixture and drizzle the dressing over the top.

Softened Broccoli with Lemon–Garlic Butter `Low Carb`

Makes 3 to 4 servings

1 bunch broccoli, cut into florets

¼ cup butter

2 cloves garlic, minced

Juice of ½ lemon

Broccoli doesn't have to be boring. The secret to making it taste amazing is to slather it in butter and drizzle some lemon juice over top. And adding some garlic certainly doesn't hurt. Sounds fattening, you say? Not really. Butter (or ghee, if you prefer) is mostly composed of short-chain fatty acids that are more readily used as fuel than stored as fat. Plus butter just tastes so good. If you're still clinging on to margarine because you think butter is bad for you, then please chuck that artificial junk. After all, you're not eating pounds of butter each week, just a little here and there. This broccoli side works really well with salmon.

1. Steam the broccoli for 5 minutes, or until the desired softness is achieved. Meanwhile, in a small skillet over medium-low heat, melt the butter. Add the garlic and cook, stirring frequently, for 2 minutes. Add the lemon juice and cook for another minute. Remove from the heat.

2. Plate the broccoli and dress it with the lemon-garlic butter from the skillet.

Herbed Smoked Salmon and Potato Hash

Makes 4 servings

2 tablespoons butter

3 large red potatoes, cut into 1" cubes

1 onion, chopped

1 green bell pepper, finely chopped

1 teaspoon sea salt

Ground black pepper

6–8 pieces smoked salmon (or 1 cooked fillet), chopped

2 tablespoons thinly sliced fresh chives

1 tablespoon chopped fresh dill

1 teaspoon chopped fresh tarragon

Juice of ½ lemon

Although this hash is technically a side dish, it can stand on its own and be a meal in and of itself. I recommend having this as a side with eggs for breakfast. Because it contains potatoes (starchy carbs), save it for your 1-Day Feasts or Regular-Cal Days. This hash also works really well as an option for a weekend brunch.

1. Melt the butter in a large nonstick skillet over medium-high heat. Add the potatoes, onion, and bell pepper. Cook, stirring often, for 10 minutes, or until golden brown. Reduce the heat to medium and continue cooking until the potatoes are tender, about 15 minutes more. Season with the salt and ground black pepper to taste.

2. When the potatoes are tender, gently fold in the salmon, chives, dill, tarragon, and lemon juice. Continue cooking until heated through, about 2 minutes more.

Garlic Cauliflower Mash

Makes 4 servings

1 teaspoon butter

3 cloves garlic, minced

1 head cauliflower, cut into florets

2 cups vegetable, chicken, or beef broth

¼ cup butter or coconut cream (the solids at the top of a can of full-fat coconut milk)

1 teaspoon sea salt

Ground black pepper

This side is a great low-carb alternative to mashed potatoes. Thus, it's perfect for your Low-Carb Days and any other time you crave creamy garlic goodness without the heaviness of mashed potatoes. It works really well as a side with any red meat dishes and even with many of the soups in this cookbook.

1. In a small pan over medium heat, melt the butter. Add the garlic and cook, stirring frequently, for 1 to 2 minutes. Set aside.

2. In a large pot over high heat, combine the cauliflower and broth. Cover and steam for 5 minutes, or until soft. Drain.

3. In a blender, combine the garlic, cauliflower, butter or coconut cream, salt, and pepper to taste. Blend for 20 seconds, or until completely smooth. Reheat if desired. This is good topped with melted butter and chives, if desired.

Garlic Swiss Chard with Raisins and Pine Nuts

Makes 2 to 3 servings

1 bunch Swiss chard

1 tablespoon coconut oil

½ medium onion, diced

¼ cup golden raisins

2 cloves garlic, minced

½ teaspoon sea salt

Ground black pepper

¼ cup toasted pine nuts

Juice of ½ lemon

2 tablespoons olive oil

Swiss chard is probably the most flavorful of the leafy green vegetables. It has a natural sweetness that makes it very approachable, even for those who don't like greens. This side dish takes Swiss chard to a whole new level, thanks to the inclusion of raisins and pine nuts—a contrasting duo that works really well together. I would serve this as a side with any fish or chicken dishes that are a little light on veggies.

1. Chop the Swiss chard, separating the leaves from the stems but retaining both. In a large skillet over medium heat, melt the coconut oil. Add the onion and chard stems and cook, stirring frequently, for 5 minutes, or until the chard stems have softened and the onions are translucent.

2. Meanwhile, in a small cup, cover the raisins with hot water. Allow them to plump and soften slightly for about 5 minutes. Drain, reserving the water.

3. Add the Swiss chard leaves and the garlic to the skillet. Season with the salt and pepper to taste and cook, stirring frequently, for 5 minutes, or until the leaves are tender. (Add a few tablespoons of the raisin water to help steam the greens.) During the last minute of cooking, stir in the raisins, pine nuts, lemon juice, and olive oil.

Blueberry and Arugula–Stuffed Avocado

Makes 2 servings

1 avocado, halved

2 cups arugula

½ cup fresh blueberries

Juice of 1 lemon

2 tablespoons olive oil

Sea salt and ground black pepper

1 tablespoon pine nuts, sliced almonds, sunflower seeds, or pumpkin seeds

Avocados are full of fat. But it's good fat, mostly monounsaturated, which has been well documented to be very good for your heart. So don't worry about avocados, okay? They're good for you. This simple side turns an avocado into a little fruit salad bowl, which can be enjoyed on its own or alongside any lighter meals in this cookbook.

On each of 2 plates, place an avocado half. Top each half with arugula and blueberries. Drizzle with the lemon juice and olive oil. Salt and pepper to taste, then sprinkle with your favorite nuts or seeds. Serve and enjoy!

Butternut Squash and Apple Skillet

Makes 2 servings

4 cups cubed butternut squash

2 tablespoons coconut oil

1 Granny Smith apple, peeled and cubed

¼ cup chopped scallions

¼ teaspoon ground nutmeg

¼ teaspoon ground cinnamon

Sea salt and ground black pepper

¼ cup toasted chopped pecans

This is a warm and soothing healthy-carb dish perfect for those cold days when you're craving some comfort food. Since it is high in starchy carbs, it's best enjoyed on your 1-Day Feast or Regular-Cal Days. It's a substantial side that can hold its own or be paired with any chicken dishes that need a little more support.

1. In a steamer, cook the squash for 10 minutes, or until tender.

2. Melt the coconut oil in a large skillet over medium-high heat. Add the steamed squash and the apple and cook for 10 minutes, or until golden brown.

3. Add the scallions, nutmeg, cinnamon, and salt and pepper to taste and cook for 2 more minutes. Top with the toasted pecans and serve with your chosen main dish.

Chickpeas in Coconut Milk

Makes 2 servings

1 can (15 ounces)
   chickpeas, rinsed and
   drained

1 tomato, chopped

¼ teaspoon ground cloves

1 clove garlic, minced

1 cup full-fat coconut milk

¾ teaspoon ground
   turmeric

Sea salt and ground black
   pepper

This is an odd side dish that you probably wouldn't think to make on your own. And that's the beauty of having a cookbook like this one that introduces new culinary experiences that might pleasantly surprise you. Chickpeas are a great source of protein, fiber, and healthy carbs, and this side dish can work well with most chicken and fish dishes. You can also enjoy the leftovers as a healthy snack when those hunger pangs hit.

In a medium saucepan over medium heat, combine the chickpeas, tomato, cloves, garlic, coconut milk, turmeric, and salt and pepper to taste. Bring to a boil, then reduce the heat and simmer, partially covered, for 20 minutes to blend the flavors.

Roasted Brussels Sprouts

Makes 4 servings

3 cups Brussels sprouts,
  outer leaves removed
  and halved

2 tablespoons butter,
  melted

Sea salt and ground black
  pepper

1 apple, peeled and diced

½ cup shelled pistachios

½ cup dried cranberries

Brussels sprouts are members of the brassica family of vegetables—possibly the most heralded group of vegetables for preventing cancer and other diseases. I love Brussels sprouts, but many people don't. If you are one of them, thankfully, this dish will make you appreciate them a little bit more. I've included dried cranberries, apple, and pistachios to bring you a wonderful medley of flavors that distracts you from the fact that you're also eating Brussels sprouts. This is a fantastic dish to have alongside red meat or chicken.

1. Preheat the oven to 400°F. Arrange the Brussels sprouts in a single layer on a large baking sheet and toss with the butter and salt and pepper to taste. Bake for 10 minutes.

2. Add the apple and pistachios to the baking sheet, distributing evenly, and bake for 5 to 10 minutes more, or to desired softness.

3. Remove from the oven, sprinkle with the dried cranberries, and serve.

BBQ Butternut Squash Steaks

Makes 3 servings

½ **large butternut squash, seeded**

2 **tablespoons coconut oil, melted**

1 **teaspoon liquid smoke**

¼ **cup raw honey or maple syrup**

1 **teaspoon garlic powder**

1 **teaspoon paprika**

1 **teaspoon chili powder**

1 **teaspoon sea salt**

2 **cups cooked wild rice**

1 **teaspoon fresh parsley for garnish**

Whether you're someone who can't live without steak, or someone who can't imagine eating steak, these southern BBQ butternut squash steaks are a must-try.

1. Preheat the oven to 400°F. Line a baking sheet with parchment paper.

2. Place the squash half on the baking sheet. Drizzle with the oil.

3. In a small bowl, stir together the liquid smoke and honey or maple syrup. Drizzle over the squash. In another small bowl, mix together the garlic powder, paprika, chili powder, and salt. Sprinkle on top of the squash.

4. Bake for 25 to 35 minutes, or until the squash is tender. Allow to cool slightly. Serve over wild rice, garnished with fresh parsley.

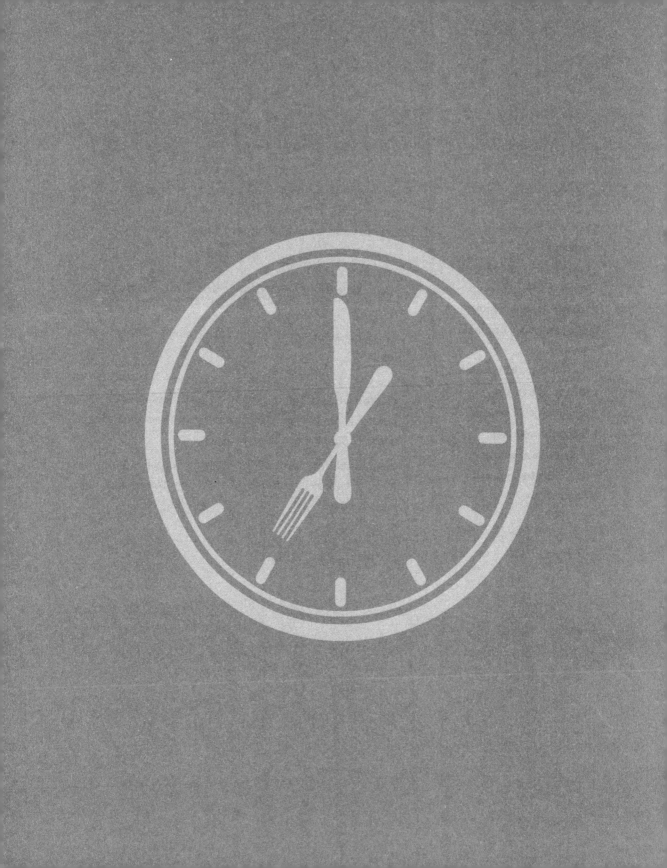

Chapter 7

Dips, Snacks, and Toppings

IN THIS SECTION you'll get easy-to-make dips, which will make eating vegetables a lot more enjoyable. You'll also get some great on-the-go snack ideas that you can turn to when those hunger pangs hit. And I'll give you some healthy alternatives to common toppings like mayonnaise and whipped cream. Some of the recipes in this book refer to these "add-ons" in their instructions, so now you know where to come for all the goods.

Hummus

Makes about 4 cups

1 can (15 ounces)
  chickpeas

3 tablespoons tahini

Juice of 1 lemon (or more
  if you like it tangy)

¼ cup olive oil

Sea salt and ground black
  pepper

Hummus is likely the most popular Middle Eastern dip that North Americans have brought into their kitchens. It's so famous that it's hard not to find numerous ready-made versions at your local grocery store. The trouble with these store-bought versions, though, is that they usually use rancid oils like canola or soybean oil instead of higher-quality olive oil. Your best bet is to make your hummus from scratch, following this recipe. Keep it in a glass container in the fridge for about a week and have it ready to go, along with some veggies (think tomatoes, cucumbers, carrots, broccoli). When you or your kids get home from a busy day, you'll avoid diving into temptations and bad snack choices.

In a food processor, combine the chickpeas, tahini, lemon juice, olive oil, and salt and pepper to taste. Blend for 20 to 30 seconds, or until smooth and creamy. If needed, add more lemon juice and/or olive oil to reach the desired consistency.

Guacamole

Makes about 4 cups

3 ripe avocados

1 small tomato, diced

¼ red onion, minced

Juice of 1 lime

1 clove garlic, minced

**¼ cup chopped fresh
  cilantro**

Who doesn't like guacamole, right? From a fat-burning perspective, I would recommend that you enjoy this guacamole with freshly cut vegetables instead of deep-fried tortilla chips. If you have leftovers that you want to keep in the fridge, then here's the trick: Keep them in an airtight glass container with plastic wrap pressed down firmly against the guacamole. The reason is that oxygen will turn the avocado brown, so you want to limit exposure to the air.

In a large bowl, combine the avocados, tomato, onion, lime juice, garlic, and cilantro. Mash with a fork until the desired chunkiness or smoothness is achieved.

Coconut Whipped Cream

Makes about 2 cups

**2 cans (14 ounces each)
full-fat coconut milk,
chilled**

1 teaspoon vanilla extract

Pinch of ground cinnamon

**1 teaspoon powdered
xylitol**

For this to work well, be sure to let the cans of coconut milk sit in the fridge for a few hours ahead of time so the fat can solidify. If you're used to eating yogurt, then this is a great nondairy substitute. And please remember, the healthy fats in coconut are very good for you—so eat to your heart's content.

Into a large bowl, scoop the thick, creamy part at the tops of the cans of coconut milk. Discard the liquid. Add the vanilla, cinnamon, and xylitol. Using an electric mixer, beat the coconut cream for 2 to 3 minutes, or until lightly fluffy.

Metabolic Mayo

Makes 2 cups

2 large eggs

**2 tablespoons lemon juice
or apple cider vinegar**

½ teaspoon Himalayan salt

**1½ cups extra light olive oil
or avocado oil**

Traditional mayonnaise is really not that good for you. It's loaded with cheap oils (like canola) and sugar that increase inflammation in your body. This recipe is simple to make and will taste just as good as, if not better than, regular mayo. The key is to use light olive oil. If you use traditional olive oil, the flavor will likely be a bit too intense for a neutral-tasting mayo. Use this mayonnaise anywhere you'd normally use mayo. It's that simple.

1. In a glass jar, such as a mason jar, combine the eggs, lemon juice or apple cider vinegar, salt, and oil. Let sit for a few seconds so that the egg settles at the bottom of the jar, underneath the oil.

2. Insert an immersion blender until it makes contact with the bottom of the jar. Blend for 30 seconds, or until the mixture emulsifies and turns into a creamy and thick concoction.

3. Store in the refrigerator in an airtight container for up to 2 weeks.

Baba Ghanoush

Makes 4 cups

1 large eggplant (about 1 pound)

2 cloves garlic, minced

2 tablespoons minced flat-leaf parsley

2 tablespoons tahini

2 tablespoons olive oil + additional for drizzling

Juice of ½ lemon

Pinch of sea salt

My dad is Moroccan, and so I've always had an affinity for North African and Middle Eastern dishes. One of my favorites is the creamy and flavorful baba ghanoush. This is a great alternative to hummus, which most people tend to gravitate toward when seeking quick-fix dips. As with hummus, you can use this as a spread or serve it alongside fresh veggies.

1. Preheat the oven to 450°F. Prick the eggplant with a fork and place it on a baking sheet lined with foil. Bake the eggplant until it is soft inside, about 20 minutes. Then let it cool.

2. Cut the eggplant in half lengthwise, drain off the liquid, and scoop the pulp into a food processor. Add the garlic, parsley, tahini, 2 tablespoons olive oil, lemon juice, and salt and process for 20 seconds, or until smooth. Transfer to a medium bowl. Drizzle with a dash of olive oil and enjoy.

Mini Meatballs

Makes 8 to 12 small
meatballs

1 large egg

**1 tablespoon Dijon
mustard**

1 clove garlic, minced

**1 tablespoon caraway
seeds**

**¼ cup minced flat-leaf
parsley**

½ teaspoon sea salt

**½ teaspoon ground black
pepper**

**2 pounds ground pork or
ground turkey**

If you want a high-protein snack that's a little more interesting than a handful of nuts, then take these Mini Meatballs with you. They're delicious, simple to make, and their protein will help you keep going for hours so you don't cave in to midafternoon cravings. As a bonus, they also make terrific hors d'oeuvres for your next dinner party.

1. Preheat the oven to 400°F and line a large baking sheet with parchment paper.

2. In a large bowl, mix the egg, mustard, garlic, caraway seeds, parsley, salt, and pepper with a fork until combined. With your hands, crumble the pork or turkey into the bowl and mix until all of the ingredients are incorporated.

3. Moisten your hands with water and shake to remove the excess. Measure a level tablespoon of the meatball mixture and roll it into a ball between your palms. Continue making meatballs until you've used all of the mixture.

4. Put the meatballs on the baking sheet, about 1" apart. Bake for 20 to 25 minutes, until golden brown and cooked through.

Kale Chips

Makes about 5 cups

1 large bunch kale leaves
   (10–12), stems removed
1 tablespoon olive oil
Sea salt and freshly
   ground black pepper

Ever get a craving for something salty? Well, instead of reaching for that bag of fattening potato chips, you can rely on these healthy, crunchy, and salty kale chips. If you're not a fan of kale, don't worry, because it actually tastes better when baked with salt and olive oil. Store (or travel with) these in an airtight container to prevent them from getting crushed.

1. Preheat the oven to 275°F. Tear the kale into bite-size pieces. In a large bowl, toss the kale leaves with the olive oil. Sprinkle the leaves with salt and pepper to taste.

2. On a baking sheet, arrange the leaves in a single layer. Bake for 30 minutes, or until crisp. Cool on a wire rack or on paper towels.

Bacon-Covered Brussels Sprouts

Low Carb, Low Cal

Makes 1 serving

2 tablespoons butter

1 cup Brussels sprouts, outer leaves and tough bases removed

Sea salt and ground black pepper

2 strips bacon

Love bacon? Not too crazy about Brussels sprouts? This simple snack solves the latter problem, thanks to the salty, fatty goodness of the bacon. You can layer these on a skewer if you like or just toss them together in a bowl. This is a great snack to take with you when you're on the go, especially if you crave salt as the day wears on.

1. In a medium skillet over medium heat, melt the butter. Add the Brussels sprouts. Season with salt and pepper to taste, then cover the skillet and cook for about 10 minutes, stirring frequently, until the Brussels sprouts have softened.

2. Meanwhile, heat a large skillet over medium heat. Add the bacon and cook for 3 minutes on each side, or until desired crispness. Cool, then chop, the bacon.

3. Combine the bacon and Brussels sprouts in a bowl or alternate them on a skewer if you're feeling adventurous.

How to Make the Best Bacon

Since bacon is mostly fat, do your best to find a brand that comes from pasture-raised or free-range pork and doesn't contain nasty fillers, preservatives, and added sugar.

To get super-crunchy bacon, the secret is to straighten it by weighing down the edges as it cooks. This works well if you decide to cook your bacon in a skillet on the stove top. However, for more of a "set it and forget it" approach and to avoid potentially getting attacked by the bacon grease that pops out of the skillet, I recommend baking your bacon in the oven. It takes a little bit longer, but the bacon ends up tasting much better, I find.

Preheat the oven to 350°F, grab a large rimmed baking sheet, and line up your bacon. Bake for 5 to 7 minutes, then flip the bacon slices. Bake until your desired level of crispness is achieved. Place the cooked bacon in a bowl lined with paper towels to absorb the excess grease. Now you're ready for the best bacon ever!

Chapter 8

Salads

I DON'T KNOW ABOUT YOU, but I grew up on some pretty boring salads—iceberg lettuce, tomatoes, and cucumbers, day in and day out—at least when I did eat salad. Nowadays, things are much different. I love salads, especially when you start getting creative with different greens and dressings. It's really a lot of fun.

As a general rule, I recommend eating at least one salad per day (except on your 1-Day Fast). It's one of the more surefire ways to ensure you get enough veggies on a regular basis. If you don't like salads, then I'm sure you'll change your mind after you try any of the salads in this section.

One more tip before we dive in: Sometimes it's smarter to make a large batch of a particular dressing and keep it stored in a mason jar in the fridge. That way, when you feel like making your next salad, half your work will be done. Give it a try.

Apple-Kale Salad with Poppy Seed Dressing Low Cal

Makes 2 to 3 servings

Dressing

3 tablespoons apple cider vinegar

1 tablespoon honey

2 teaspoons Dijon mustard

1 teaspoon poppy seeds

1 teaspoon sea salt

½ teaspoon ground black pepper

2 tablespoons olive oil

¼ cup minced red onion (about ¼ medium onion)

Salad

1 pound flat-leaf kale (about 2 bunches), ribs and stems removed

2 medium Granny Smith or Fuji apples

Apple and kale make a wonderful pair. The tart sweetness of the apple balances kale's natural bite. And when you top both with the poppy seed dressing, you're in for a salad that you can turn to over and over again. This salad is super easy to make, and here's a tip: Make plenty of the poppy seed dressing and keep it in a mason jar in the fridge for easy access the next time you make this salad. It will keep for 2 weeks.

1. *To make the dressing:* In a large bowl, whisk together the vinegar, honey, mustard, poppy seeds, salt, and pepper. While whisking constantly, slowly add the oil until all of it is incorporated. Add the onion, stir to combine, and set aside.

2. *To make the salad:* Arrange the kale leaves into stacks. Slice each stack crosswise into ¼" ribbons. Add to the bowl with the dressing.

3. Core the apples and julienne them (cut them into 1½"-long matchsticks). Add them to the bowl. Toss to combine the apple and kale with the dressing. Let rest for 5 minutes for the flavors to blend, then serve.

Potato Pesto Salad

Makes 4 servings

1½ pounds baby potatoes

1½ cups packed fresh basil leaves

1 cup baby spinach

⅓ cup chopped walnuts + additional for serving

¼ teaspoon lemon peel

Juice of 1 lemon

1 clove garlic

½ teaspoon sea salt

¼ teaspoon ground black pepper

3 tablespoons olive oil

1 tablespoon chopped fresh chives

If you read *The All-Day Fat-Burning Diet,* then you know that cooked, then cooled, potatoes can actually help you lose weight and better your health. How? Because they are high in resistant starch—a type of starch that resists digestion and serves as fuel for the good bacteria in your gut. Resistant starch has been shown to improve insulin sensitivity and even reduce fat throughout the body. So yes, this cold potato salad is a fat-burning salad. Since it's cold, you can keep it for several days in the fridge and grab a few bites when you're pressed for time or just feel like getting your potato fix.

1. In a large pot of boiling salted water, cook the potatoes until slightly tender, about 12 to 15 minutes. Drain, reserving about 2 tablespoons of the cooking liquid. Submerge the potatoes in a bowl of ice water for 5 minutes, then drain. Refrigerate the potatoes for at least 1 hour to increase their resistant starch level.

2. Meanwhile, in a food processor, pulse together the basil, spinach, ⅓ cup walnuts, lemon peel and juice, garlic, salt, pepper, and oil.

3. Once the potatoes are cold, toss them with the pesto. Top with the chives and a few walnut pieces, and serve.

Shaved Carrot, Beet, and Pear Salad

Makes 4 servings

Dressing

2 tablespoons olive oil

1 tablespoon minced shallots

½ tablespoon apple cider vinegar

1 teaspoon sea salt

½ teaspoon ground black pepper

Salad

1 large beet, shaved with a mandoline or vegetable peeler

2 large carrots, also shaved

1 large Bosc pear, sliced

1 scallion, thinly sliced

1 rib celery, thinly sliced

2 cups arugula

This is a beautiful-looking salad with an array of colors, which is a good indication that it packs some serious anti-inflammatory benefits. And it doesn't hurt that it tastes darn good as well. It's a light salad that is perfectly suited to go alongside any other dish or to be enjoyed on its own, especially on your Low-Cal Days.

1. *To make the dressing:* In a small bowl, stir together the oil, shallots, vinegar, salt, and pepper. Set aside.

2. *To make the salad:* In a large bowl, combine the beet and carrot shavings, pear, scallion, celery, and arugula. Add the dressing, toss well, and plate.

Quinoa, Kale, and Currant Salad

Makes 4 servings

2 cups quinoa

3 cups water

3 cups chopped kale, ribs and stems removed

2 tablespoons pine nuts

2 tablespoons currants or raisins

Juice of ½ lemon

1 tablespoon olive oil

1 teaspoon sea salt

½ teaspoon ground black pepper

Quinoa is a gluten-free grain rich with protein and nutrients. It's very versatile and can be enjoyed in a variety of forms. In this salad, we're pairing it with the supergreen—kale—pine nuts, and a touch of currants. The result is a flavorful salad that can be enjoyed on its own. It also pairs nicely with any lighter fish, such as sole or cod.

1. In a large pot over medium-high heat, combine the quinoa and water. Bring to a boil. Cover, reduce the heat to low, and simmer until the quinoa is tender, about 15 minutes.

2. Place the chopped kale on top of the quinoa, cover, and steam the kale for 5 minutes. Add the pine nuts, currants or raisins, lemon juice, oil, salt, and pepper. Mix well. Serve warm or cold.

Tasty Thai Salad

Makes 2 servings

Salad

1 zucchini, spiralized

1 carrot, spiralized

½ beet, spiralized

⅛ head red cabbage, sliced

2 scallions, chopped

½ cup chopped fresh cilantro

Dressing

1 teaspoon sunflower seed butter or organic peanut butter

1 teaspoon water

Juice of ½ lime

½ teaspoon coconut aminos or tamari

2 tablespoons minced fresh cilantro

½ clove garlic, minced

This salad was inspired by one of my favorite Asian fusion restaurants in Toronto. This version does a pretty good job of mimicking the memories I have of the 18-ingredient salad at that restaurant. Each bite tastes like a fireworks show of complementary flavors going off in your mouth. You can enjoy it on its own for lunch (it's perfect for a Low-Carb Day or Low-Cal Day) or with any of your other mains. (If you don't have a spiralizer, you can use either a cheese grater or a vegetable peeler to prepare the zucchini, carrot, and beet.)

1. *To make the salad:* In a large bowl, combine the zucchini, carrot, beet, cabbage, scallions, and cilantro.

2. *To make the dressing:* In a blender, combine the sunflower seed butter or peanut butter, water, lime juice, coconut aminos or tamari, cilantro, and garlic. Blend until smooth, about 30 seconds.

3. Pour the dressing over the salad, mix well, and serve.

Kale and Avocado Teaser Caesar Salad

Low Carb

Makes 2 servings

Creamy Dressing

1½ tablespoons almond butter

1 tablespoon apple cider vinegar

2 tablespoons olive oil

½ teaspoon maple syrup

½ teaspoon coconut aminos or tamari

½ clove garlic

Juice of 1 lemon

1 tablespoon water

1 teaspoon sea salt

½ teaspoon ground black pepper

Salad

1 bunch kale, ribs and stems removed, chopped

2 scallions, diced

¼ cup slivered almonds

1 avocado, sliced

When I go to an Italian restaurant, I usually order a Caesar salad as a starter, assuming it's been made from scratch without all that fake Caesar dressing. Blindfold yourself and take a few bites of this kale and avocado version and you won't be able to tell that it's not a traditional Caesar dressing. The good news is that you can once again enjoy a Caesar-like salad without worrying about fake dressings that pack on the pounds. This is made from fresh, wholesome ingredients that do your body good.

1. *To make the dressing:* In a blender, combine the almond butter, vinegar, oil, maple syrup, coconut aminos or tamari, garlic, lemon juice, water, salt, and pepper. Blend until creamy, about 20 seconds.

2. *To make the salad:* In a large bowl, mix together the kale, scallions, almonds, and dressing. Top with the avocado and serve.

Kaleslaw

Makes 4 servings

Juice of ½ lemon

1 tablespoon apple cider
vinegar

2 tablespoons olive oil

1 clove garlic, minced

1 teaspoon sea salt

½ teaspoon ground black
pepper

4 cups thinly sliced kale,
ribs and stems removed

4 cups shredded cabbage

1 red bell pepper, thinly
sliced

½ apple, cored and thinly
sliced

This is a delicious salad that plays on the classic coleslaw concept. However, this version is actually good for you and not loaded with mayonnaise and rancid oils. I would pair it with a red meat or a denser, legume-based dish. It's also perfect for both Low-Carb Days and Low-Cal Days.

In a large bowl, whisk together the lemon juice, vinegar, oil, garlic, salt, and pepper. Stir in the kale, cabbage, red pepper, and apple. Toss to combine. Cover and refrigerate for at least 4 hours before serving.

How to Keep Your Greens Crisp Longer

There's nothing worse than greens that get slimy and wilted shortly after you buy them. So here's how to store them in your fridge to help them live fresh and crisp for several days longer.

Wash and dry the leaves and stem them, if necessary (think kale). Pat them dry with a paper towel.

Line a plastic storage container with paper towels, then dump the greens in an even layer on top, and covered them with another layer of paper towel before locking down the lid. The paper towels will help absorb excess moisture from the greens and keep them from getting slimy, and the sealed container keeps excess air from circulating in and out, thus slowing the wilting process. Following these steps should make your greens last for 10 to 14 days in the fridge.

Lentilicious Salad

Makes 2 servings

1½ cups water

1½ cups vegetable stock

1 cup green lentils

1 shallot, minced

2 tablespoons olive oil

Juice of ½ lemon

½ teaspoon lemon peel

1 teaspoon sea salt

½ teaspoon ground black pepper

½ head Boston lettuce, thinly sliced

¼ head radicchio, thinly sliced

1 rib celery, thinly sliced

1 apple, sliced

2 tablespoons dried cranberries

¼ cup walnuts

Lentils are one of the highest sources of protein in our food supply. They're also packed with fiber and healthy carbs, making them a complete meal even by themselves. This salad is based on lentils but brought to life with a myriad of flavors that I'm sure you'll enjoy. Since this is a heartier salad, you can have it as a meal all by itself or pair it with a lighter main or soup.

1. In a medium pot over high heat, combine the water, stock, and lentils. Bring to a boil, cover tightly, reduce the heat to medium-low, and simmer until the lentils are tender, about 15 to 20 minutes. Remove from the burner and let cool.

2. Meanwhile, in a large bowl, whisk together the shallot, oil, lemon juice and peel, salt, and pepper. Add the cooled lentils, lettuce, radicchio, celery, apple, cranberries, and walnuts. Toss to combine, then serve.

Spinach, Jicama, and Apple Salad

Salad

6 cups baby spinach

1 apple, sliced

**½ jicama, julienned
(substitute ½ fennel bulb
if jicama is unavailable)**

¼ cup walnuts

1 avocado, cubed

Dressing

2 tablespoons olive oil

**2 tablespoons apple cider
vinegar**

1 teaspoon honey

2 teaspoons Dijon mustard

½ clove garlic, minced

1 teaspoon sea salt

**½ teaspoon ground black
pepper**

Jicama is also known as the "Mexican turnip." It's one of my favorite root vegetables. Its inside is creamy white and it has a crisp texture that resembles that of raw potato or pear, yet its flavor is sweet and starchy, reminiscent of some apples. I find that it tastes best raw, especially when julienned and paired with greens and apple. That's what you'll find in this delicious salad. Feel free to pair it with any main dish on any day other than your Low-Carb Days.

1. *To make the salad:* In a large bowl, combine the spinach, apple, jicama, walnuts, and avocado.

2. *To make the dressing:* In a smaller bowl, whisk together the oil, vinegar, honey, mustard, garlic, salt, and pepper. Pour over the salad, toss, and serve.

Cooled Potato, Beet, and Lentil Salad

Feast Approved

Makes 2 to 3 servings

3 cups water

1 cup red lentils

2 medium beets

10 small red potatoes

½ small red onion, sliced

1 handful fresh cilantro, chopped

1 tablespoon apple cider vinegar

2 tablespoons olive oil

1 teaspoon sea salt

Ground black pepper

Here's another take on the good old cooled potato salad. This is a hearty dish that features some pretty heavy-duty starchy carbs, so I'd reserve this one for a 1-Day Feast or Regular-Cal Day. It can stand on its own or be paired with a light soup or lighter main.

1. Into a medium pot over high heat, pour the water. Add the lentils. Bring to a boil, cover, reduce the heat to medium-low, and simmer until the lentils are tender, about 15 minutes.

2. Meanwhile, in a large pot, place the whole, unpeeled beets and potatoes. Add enough cold water so that they're fully submerged. Bring to a boil over high heat, then reduce the heat to medium-low and simmer for about 20 minutes, or until a fork will penetrate both the beets and potatoes with ease.

3. Place the pot of beets and potatoes under running cold water. Let cool for 3 to 5 minutes, then peel the beets. Cut them and the potatoes into quarter-size pieces.

4. In a large bowl, combine the beets, potatoes, lentils, and red onion. Refrigerate for at least 2 hours, or overnight.

5. When cooled, add the cilantro, vinegar, oil, salt, and pepper to taste. Combine well and serve.

Swiss Chard, Bean, and Bacon Tahini Salad

Makes 2 to 3 servings

Salad

1 head Swiss chard (about 10 leaves), stemmed and chopped

1 can (15 ounces) cannellini beans, rinsed and drained

2 strips crispy cooked bacon, chopped

Tahini Dressing

⅓ cup tahini

1 clove garlic, minced

Juice of 1 lemon

2 tablespoons olive oil

1 tablespoon chopped parsley

1 teaspoon sea salt

Ground black pepper

Just wait until you try this salad. That's all I can say about this one. The odd combination of these three ingredients, topped with a delicious tahini dressing, will pleasantly surprise you. Plus, who doesn't love bacon, right? Perfect alongside any meat dish and for any day other than your Low-Carb Days.

1. *To make the salad:* In a large bowl, combine the Swiss chard, beans, and bacon. Set aside.

2. *To make the dressing:* In a smaller bowl, whisk together the tahini, garlic, lemon juice, oil, parsley, salt, and pepper to taste. Add a splash or two of hot water to thin the dressing, until it is pourable.

3. Pour the dressing over the salad, mix well, and serve.

Wilted Spinach, Quinoa, and Olive Salad

Makes 2 servings

2 cups vegetable broth

1 cup quinoa

2 tablespoons olive oil

1 clove garlic, minced

½ teaspoon crushed red-
   pepper flakes

1 cup diced mushrooms

½ cup diced yellow bell
   pepper

4 cups baby spinach

½ cup chopped fresh basil

¼ cup chopped sun-dried
   tomatoes

½ cup kalamata olives,
   pitted

Juice of ½ lemon

1 teaspoon sea salt

Ground black pepper

Looking at the title of this recipe, you'd think it was something out of Popeye and Olive's kitchen. In all seriousness, this salad combines the nutrient-rich powers of spinach, quinoa, and olives. Olives are rich in monounsaturated fats, which is part of the reason why the Mediterranean diet tends to be healthier for your heart and waistline. Enjoy this salad on any day, including your Low-Carb Days. (The small amount of quinoa won't put you over the net carb threshold for the day, so don't worry.)

1. In a medium pot over high heat, combine the broth and quinoa. Bring to a boil. Cover, reduce the heat to low, and simmer until the quinoa is tender and fluffy, about 15 minutes. Set aside to cool.

2. Meanwhile, in a large skillet over medium-low heat, place the oil. Add the garlic and red-pepper flakes and cook for about 30 seconds. Add the mushrooms and yellow pepper. Cook for 5 minutes, or until the mushrooms are soft. Reduce the heat to low and add the spinach and basil. Stir for 5 minutes, or until the spinach is wilted.

3. Finally, add the quinoa, tomatoes, olives, and lemon juice. Stir well. Season with the salt and ground black pepper to taste.

Potato and Lentil Protein Salad

Feast Approved

Makes 4 servings

2 pounds red potatoes

2 scallions, chopped

2 dill pickles, chopped

**1 handful fresh dillweed,
   chopped**

½ cup cooked lentils

**3–4 tablespoons
   Metabolic Mayo
   (page 131)**

**1 tablespoon Dijon
   mustard**

**Sea salt and ground black
   pepper**

We've discussed the health benefits of cold potatoes, so no need to beat a dead horse. This salad combines cooled potatoes and protein-rich lentils, along with flavor enhancers like pickles and Metabolic Mayo. I know you'll appreciate the end result. This is another great salad for leftovers, as it will keep for at least a week in the fridge. Just save the last step—adding the mayo and mustard to the potatoes—until you're ready to serve. Perfect for any day other than your Low-Carb Days.

1. Place the potatoes in a large pot and cover them with water. Bring to a boil over medium-high heat, reduce the heat to medium-low, and simmer for 5 to 7 minutes, or just until the potatoes can be pierced with a fork. Strain the potatoes and run them under cold water for 2 minutes, then set aside. Once cooled enough, cut the potatoes into halves or quarters.

2. Meanwhile, in a large bowl, stir together the scallions, pickles, dill, and lentils. Add the potatoes, Metabolic Mayo to taste, and mustard. Season to taste with salt and pepper. Stir to coat and chill in the refrigerator for 1 to 2 hours. Serve cold.

Citrus and Avocado Salad

Makes 2 servings

2 small oranges, peeled and sliced

3 tablespoons olive oil

1 tablespoon apple cider vinegar or balsamic vinegar

1 tablespoon chopped fresh basil

Sea salt and freshly ground black pepper

4 cups baby spinach

¼ bulb fennel, thinly sliced

1 avocado, sliced

1 scallion, chopped

Avocado works really well when paired with almost any tropical fruit, especially citrus fruits. In this salad, you'll experience the wonderful flavors and textures of oranges and avocado, along with a hint of basil that elevates this salad to a whole other level. This is a great afternoon salad on a warm summer's day and can be enjoyed on any day other than your Low-Carb Days.

1. In a medium bowl, toss the oranges with the oil, vinegar, basil, and salt and pepper to taste. Let the mixture sit for at least 5 minutes.

2. In a large serving bowl, combine the spinach, fennel, avocado, and scallion. Top with the orange and dressing mixture, toss well, and serve.

Curried Chickpea Salad

Makes 2 to 3 servings

1 teaspoon apple cider
vinegar

1 tablespoon lemon juice

2 tablespoons olive oil

1 tablespoon curry powder

1 teaspoon maple syrup

Sea salt and ground black
pepper

1 can (15 ounces)
chickpeas, rinsed and
drained

2 ribs celery, diced

½ red onion, sliced

¼ cup chopped parsley

1 Granny Smith apple,
peeled and diced

¼ cup raisins

½ head romaine lettuce,
chopped

Chickpeas taste amazing when they've been combined with curry. This salad brings that flavor to you alongside the crisp textures of celery and apple, with a hint of raisiny sweetness. If you're looking for a new way to get more health-promoting legumes into your diet, then this salad could very well become a staple for you. Enjoy it on its own or alongside a soup on any day other than your Low-Carb Days.

1. In a large bowl, whisk together the vinegar, lemon juice, oil, curry powder, maple syrup, and salt and pepper to taste.

2. Add the chickpeas, celery, onion, parsley, apple, raisins, and lettuce. Toss to combine.

Spicy Garlic Oven-Roasted Chickpeas

2 cans (15 ounces) chickpeas, rinsed and drained

¼ cup olive oil

1 teaspoon sea salt, divided + additional to taste

½ teaspoon chili powder

½ teaspoon ground cumin

¾ teaspoon paprika

¾ teaspoon garlic powder

½ teaspoon onion powder

¼–½ teaspoon ground red pepper

These crunchy chickpeas will easily replace less-healthy snacks in your repertoire.

1. Preheat the oven to 425°F. Line a baking sheet with parchment paper.

2. Place the chickpeas in a strainer lined with a paper towel. Allow to air-dry for 10 to 15 minutes.

3. Place the chickpeas on the baking sheet. Drizzle with the oil and stir to coat. Sprinkle with ½ teaspoon of the salt. Bake, stirring every 5 minutes, for 20 to 25 minutes, or until golden brown. (Some of the chickpeas may start popping. This is a good sign that they're properly crisping.)

4. Meanwhile, in a large bowl, stir together the remaining ½ teaspoon salt, chili powder, cumin, paprika, garlic powder, onion powder, and red pepper. Toss the hot chickpeas in the spice mixture. Add additional salt to taste, if desired. Serve and enjoy immediately.

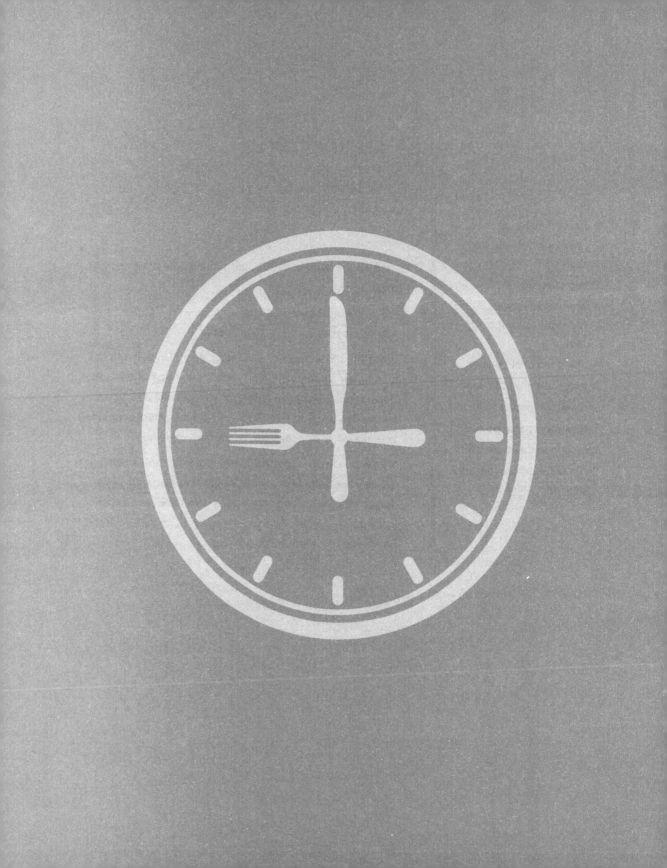

Chapter 9

Bowls and Quick-Fix Lunches

LUNCHTIME CAN GET PRETTY HECTIC. Unless you're at home with nothing to do, it's very unlikely that you'll have time to put together an elaborate meal. That's why meal bowls are awesome. They're an easy, versatile, and nutritious way to think about lunch—or even dinner. Putting together a meal bowl is easy, and I've assembled some tips and inspiring ideas to make it even easier.

All of these bowls are vegan, so they're perfect for those looking for delicious and filling ways to get more plant foods into their diet. You'll find a combination of rice-based, noodle-based, and legume-based bowls with a variety of toppings and unique dressings to make the flavors really pop. I've also put together some simple combinations with collard rolls and "zoodles" (zucchini noodles) that are perfect for quick-fix lunches. Dig in!

Vermicelli Garden Bowl

Makes 2 servings

¼ pound vermicelli noodles

1 tablespoon coconut oil

½ onion, sliced

2 cloves garlic, minced

2 cups baby spinach

1 carrot, julienned

½ red bell pepper, julienned

1 cup stemmed, chopped shiitake mushrooms

1 tablespoon sesame oil

1 tablespoon coconut aminos or tamari

1 teaspoon sea salt

Ground black pepper

Asian vermicelli noodles are derived from rice and have a light, waxy texture. Because of their carb content, I would reserve this bowl for any day other than your Low-Carb Days. On its own, this is a fairly light dish, so it's perfect for lunch on a Low-Cal Day. If you're looking for a light vegan lunch option, then this is great.

1. Bring a large pot of salted water to a boil over high heat. Add the vermicelli, reduce the heat, and simmer until tender, about 5 minutes. Drain and rinse the noodles and set them aside.

2. Meanwhile, in a wok or large saucepan over medium heat, melt the coconut oil. Add the onion and cook, stirring frequently, for 3 minutes, or until golden. Add the garlic and spinach and cook for 1 minute. Add the carrot, red pepper, mushrooms, sesame oil, coconut aminos or tamari, salt, and ground black pepper to taste. Cook, stirring frequently, for another 1 to 2 minutes, until the vegetables are tender-crisp.

3. Pour the noodles over the veggies in the saucepan and stir to combine. Remove from the heat and serve.

Rainbow Rice Bowl

Makes 2 servings

1 cup brown rice

2 handfuls kale, ribs and
stems removed

2 cups baby spinach

Juice of 1 lemon

2 tablespoons olive oil

2 tablespoons tahini

1 clove garlic, minced

1 tablespoon minced
scallion

1 teaspoon sea salt

½ teaspoon ground black
pepper

½ red bell pepper,
julienned

½ orange bell pepper,
julienned

1 avocado, sliced

As its name implies, this bowl is loaded with colors, which is always a good sign that what you're about to eat is full of health-promoting nutrients. This bowl is quite substantial and, if you have it for lunch, will likely keep you satisfied well beyond dinner. Because of its rice content, I would reserve this for any day other than your Low-Carb Days.

1. Cook the rice according to package instructions. Meanwhile, in a steamer over high heat, cook the kale and spinach for 5 to 7 minutes, until slightly wilted.

2. In a small bowl, whisk together the lemon juice, oil, tahini, garlic, scallion, salt, and pepper.

3. Place the rice in a serving bowl. Top it with the wilted kale and spinach, bell peppers, and avocado. Drizzle the dressing over the top and serve.

Greens and Orange over Rice

Makes 2 servings

Rice Bowl

1 cup brown rice

½ bulb fennel, thinly shaved

1 cup watercress

1 cup baby spinach

1 orange, peeled and segmented

¼ red onion, thinly sliced

1 avocado, sliced

¼ cup chopped walnuts

Dressing

2 tablespoons olive oil

1 tablespoon apple cider vinegar

2 tablespoons freshly squeezed orange juice

2 tablespoons minced shallots

1 teaspoon sea salt

½ teaspoon ground black pepper

This is a fresh take on the traditional rice bowl, thanks to its inclusion of orange, watercress, and fennel—three ingredients that work really well together and have a fresh feel to them. The dressing for this bowl is also remarkably good, which makes a seemingly plain rice bowl pack so much flavor. Enjoy this rice bowl on any day other than your Low-Carb Days.

1. *To make the bowl:* Cook the rice according to package instructions. Place the cooked rice in a serving bowl. Top with the fennel, watercress, spinach, orange segments, onion, avocado, and walnuts.

2. *To make the dressing:* In a small bowl, whisk together the oil, vinegar, orange juice, shallots, salt, and pepper. Drizzle the dressing over the top of the rice bowl.

Green Chickpea Tahini Bowl

Makes 2 servings

Chickpea Bowl

½ bunch asparagus (about 10 pieces), trimmed

1 cup halved cherry tomatoes

1 tablespoon coconut oil, melted

1 teaspoon sea salt

½ teaspoon ground black pepper

2 big handfuls kale, ribs and stems removed

1 can (15 ounces) chickpeas, rinsed well and drained

½ teaspoon ground cumin

½ teaspoon ground cinnamon

½ teaspoon chili powder

2 tablespoons olive oil

1 avocado, sliced

Tahini Sauce

¼ cup tahini

1 teaspoon maple syrup

Juice of ½ lemon

1 clove garlic, minced

1–2 tablespoons hot water

If you're tired of rice bowls and want something unique, then give this chickpea bowl a shot. The chickpeas hold the flavor of the spices, and the entire bowl is dressed in a delicious tahini sauce. Tahini, a paste made from sesame seeds, is rich in calcium, so it provides a mineral boost along with its great flavor. Enjoy this bowl on any day other than your Low-Carb Days.

1. *To make the bowl:* Preheat the oven to 400°F. Place the asparagus and tomatoes on a roasting pan and toss with the melted coconut oil, salt, and pepper. Roast for 15 to 20 minutes. Remove from the oven and chop the asparagus into thirds. Meanwhile, in a steamer over high heat, cook the kale for 5 minutes.

2. In a large skillet over medium heat, combine the chickpeas with the cumin, cinnamon, and chili powder. Mix well. Add the olive oil and cook, stirring frequently, until lightly browned, 6 to 8 minutes. Remove from the heat and set aside.

3. *To make the sauce:* In a medium bowl, whisk together the tahini, maple syrup, lemon juice, and garlic. Add enough hot water to form a pourable sauce.

4. To serve, divide the asparagus, tomatoes, kale, and chickpea mixture between 2 bowls. Top with the Tahini Sauce and sliced avocado, and enjoy.

Mashed Split Pea and Avocado Bowl

Makes 2 servings

1 tablespoon coconut oil

1 leek, thinly sliced

2 cloves garlic, minced

1 cup yellow split peas

3 cups vegetable broth

1 tablespoon diced chives

1 teaspoon crushed or chopped fresh rosemary

1 teaspoon sea salt

Freshly ground black pepper

1 cup quartered cherry tomatoes

1 ripe avocado, sliced

Split peas are one of the highest-protein foods on the planet. Their protein is so complete and rich in amino acids that pea protein is one of the most sought-after vegan protein powders on the market. This bowl gives you a whopping serving of protein and healthy fats, flavored with aromatic herbs. A wonderful vegan bowl for any day other than your Low-Carb Days.

1. In a large pot over medium heat, melt the coconut oil. Add the leek and garlic and cook, stirring frequently, for 2 minutes, or until softened.

2. Add the split peas and broth, increase the heat to medium-high, and bring to a rapid simmer. Reduce the heat to medium-low, cover, and simmer for 50 minutes, stirring occasionally, until the split peas are tender and mushy and most of the liquid has been absorbed. The finished split peas should be creamy and resemble mashed potatoes. If they aren't, add water and stir until the peas break down and the water is absorbed.

3. Remove from the heat and stir in the chives, rosemary, sea salt, and black pepper to taste. Divide between 2 bowls and top with the cherry tomatoes and avocado slices.

On-the-Go Green Lunch Bowls

Here are 10 more simple bowl ideas that you can throw together for a healthy lunch at work or even at home. Simply find the flavor combinations that most appeal to you and go nuts. To keep these bowls from getting soggy, pack your greens, toppings, and dressings in separate airtight containers and combine them when you're ready to eat. I haven't included quantities to give you room to play around with how much of each ingredient you'd like, but each bowl will likely consist of about 2 servings.

Here's how to make them.

1. Start with a bowl. Add a few handfuls of your favorite leafy greens, such as baby kale, spinach, and/or chopped Swiss chard.

2. Toss in one of the following 10 topping and dressing combos for a fantastic and healthy lunch. Now you're all set!

THAI CHICKEN BOWL

Topping: Shredded cooked chicken breast, chopped carrots, edamame, scallions, chopped fresh cilantro, and peanuts

Dressing: 2 tablespoons sweet chili sauce, 1 tablespoon rice wine vinegar, 1 tablespoon canned coconut milk, ½ tablespoon brown sugar, 1 teaspoon melted creamy peanut butter, 1 minced clove garlic, juice of ½ lime, ⅛ teaspoon ground ginger

CUBAN BOWL

Topping: Black beans, roasted sweet potato, roasted cauliflower, chopped fresh cilantro and scallions

Dressing: 3 tablespoons fresh lime juice, 2 tablespoons olive oil, 1 minced clove garlic, 1 teaspoon ground cumin, 1 teaspoon pure maple syrup, ½ teaspoon sea salt

(continued)

ASIAN PEANUT BOWL

Topping: Diced red bell pepper, diced carrot, shredded cabbage, edamame, chopped scallions

Dressing: ¼ cup creamy peanut butter, 2 tablespoons soy sauce, 1 tablespoon water, 1 tablespoon honey, 1 tablespoon rice wine vinegar, 1 teaspoon grated fresh ginger, 1 teaspoon sesame oil, 1 minced clove garlic

TROPICAL BOWL

Topping: Diced mango, diced red bell pepper, diced carrots, cashews, chopped cilantro

Dressing: ¼ cup full-fat coconut milk, 1 tablespoon white wine vinegar, 1 teaspoon lime peel, 1 teaspoon brown sugar, juice of ½ lime

CHIPOTLE CHICKEN BOWL

Topping: Chopped seasoned and grilled chicken, black beans, chopped avocado, chopped fresh cilantro, chopped tomato

Dressing: Juice of 1 lime, 1 tablespoon olive oil, ½ tablespoon honey

ROASTED VEGGIE BOWL

Topping: Roasted red bell peppers, roasted zucchini, roasted mushrooms, chopped walnuts

Dressing: Juice of 1 lemon, 1 tablespoon olive oil, ½ cup chopped parsley, 1 minced clove garlic, salt and ground black pepper

NICOISE SALAD BOWL

Topping: Canned tuna, chopped hard-cooked egg, steamed green beans, sliced roasted potato, sliced roasted beets, black olives

Dressing: 1 tablespoon lemon juice, 2 tablespoons olive oil, ½ teaspoon dried basil, ¼ teaspoon ground thyme, ¼ teaspoon dried oregano, ½ teaspoon Dijon mustard, salt and ground black pepper

SWEET AND SOUR CASHEW-BROCCOLI BOWL

Topping: Steamed broccoli, cashews, chopped scallions

Dressing: 1 tablespoon coconut aminos, ½ teaspoon sesame oil, 1 tablespoon rice wine vinegar, 1 minced clove garlic, 1 tablespoon honey

CHICKEN PESTO BOWL

Topping: Grilled chicken, diced tomato

Dressing: Pesto sauce

MISO BOWL

Topping: Roasted sweet potato, roasted beets, chopped scallions, black beans

Dressing: 1 tablespoon white miso paste, 1 tablespoon tahini, $\frac{1}{2}$ tablespoon rice wine vinegar, $\frac{1}{4}$ cup water

Raw Collard Wraps

Collard greens are a popular leafy green vegetable for creating wraps, rolls, and even "tacos." Collard leaves are thick enough to hold a good number of ingredients, which makes them a perfect alternative to bread and wheat-based wraps, and these quick-fix lunches are super simple to throw together, easy to take to work, and a great way to load up on nutrition. Just rinse and dry a good-size collard leaf, fill it with any of the following ingredient combos, and fold or wrap. I again haven't included quantities to give you room to play around with how much of each ingredient you'd like.

Here are 10 great combos, enough for 2 workweeks.

GOOD GODDESS WRAP

Hummus, tomatoes, fresh basil, balsamic vinegar

VEGAN MEDITERRANEAN WRAP

Cherry tomatoes, kalamata olives, chickpeas, sliced red onion, olive oil and lemon juice

VEGAN ANTIPASTI WRAP

Sliced red onion, kalamata olives, cannellini beans, olive oil and lemon juice

APPLE SALAD WRAP

Diced apples, chopped walnuts, chopped celery, olive oil or Metabolic Mayo (page 131)

VEGAN CHILI WRAP

Cannellini beans, diced onion, diced tomatoes, ground cumin, chili powder

GUACAMOLE WRAP

Mashed avocado, diced red onion, diced tomatoes, lime juice

CHICKEN AND RICE WRAP

Diced cooked chicken, brown rice, ground cumin, ground turmeric

RICE AND BEANS WRAP

Brown rice, cannellini beans, olive oil and balsamic vinegar

AUTUMN HARVEST WRAP

Chopped cooked butternut squash, chopped apples, brown rice

BACON AND EGG WRAP

Chopped hard-cooked egg, chopped bacon, chopped scallions, Metabolic Mayo (page 131)

Zippy Zoodles

If you're tired of bowls, wraps, and leftovers for lunch, try a bowl of fresh zoodles instead. You'll cut out refined grains while getting a nutritious and tasty lunch. Zoodles are zucchini spirals made with a julienne peeler or a spiralizer, and they're perfect for paleo, vegan, and gluten-free diets. These are great for your Low-Carb Days and your Low-Cal Days.

1. Peel a medium zucchini. Using a vegetable peeler or julienne peeler, cut it into long, spaghetti-like strands. You can also use a spiralizer, which turns a zucchini and many other veggies into spaghetti-like strands in seconds.

2. You can use your zoodles raw or lightly stir-fry them. Next, we'll load on some yummy toppings!

3. Place your zoodles in a bowl and add one of the following 10 delicious topping mixtures.

PESTO ZOODLES

Chopped fresh basil, pine nuts, minced garlic, olive oil, salt and ground black pepper

SESAME ZOODLES

Chopped scallions, soy sauce, rice wine vinegar, sesame oil, peanut butter, and minced garlic

CHOW MEIN ZOODLES

Cooked ground pork, shaved carrots, fish sauce, sesame oil, grated fresh ginger, salt

MEDITERRANEAN ZOODLES

Cherry tomatoes, artichoke hearts, kalamata olives, red wine vinegar, olive oil, salt, goat cheese (optional)

RAW TOMATO SAUCE ZOODLES

Chopped tomatoes, sun-dried tomatoes, minced garlic, olive oil, salt and ground black pepper

COCONUT CURRY ZOODLES

Snap peas, diced carrots, green curry paste, coconut milk, fish sauce, and coconut aminos

PAD THAI ZOODLES

Hard-cooked egg, chopped scallions, julienned carrots, lime juice, fish sauce, coconut aminos, and chili powder

SHRIMP SCAMPI ZOODLES

Cooked shrimp, cherry tomatoes, minced garlic, lemon juice, salt and ground black pepper

CHICKEN ZOODLE SOUP

Chopped cooked chicken, chicken broth, chopped onion, chopped carrots, minced garlic, salt and ground black pepper

CREAMY AVOCADO ZOODLES

Sliced avocado, sliced cucumbers, minced garlic, coconut milk, chopped fresh basil, salt and ground black pepper

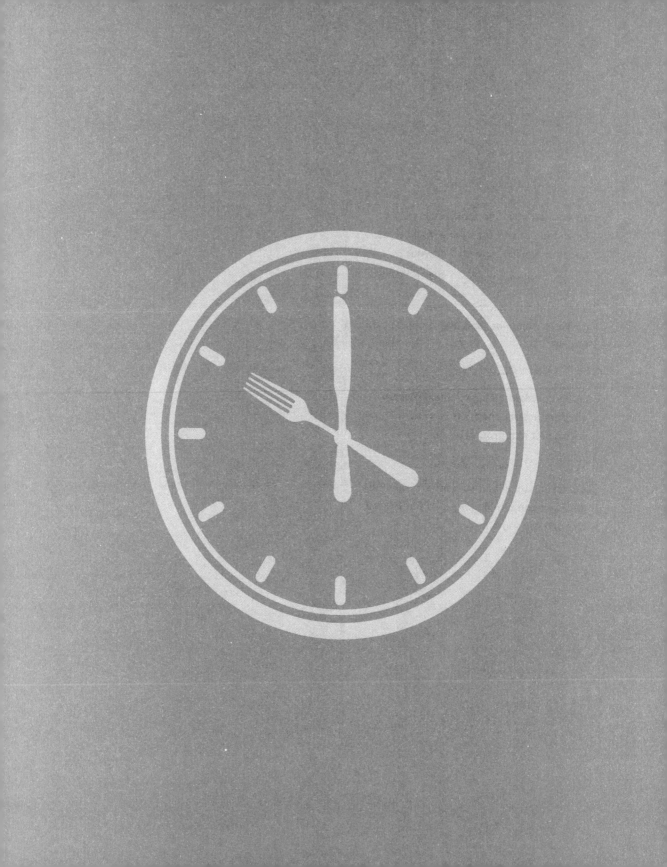

Chapter 10

Soups

SOUPS ARE LIKE WARM SMOOTHIES, if you ask me. In my house, we make soups and stews weekly because they're such an easy way to feed our kids a good variety of wholesome foods in a convenient format. Plus, when you make a good amount, you've got leftovers for days, which can easily be reheated when you're short on time and still want great nutrition.

Many of the soups in this section feature legumes like chickpeas, lentils, and beans as a way of giving you some more protein and fiber, both of which are extremely important for keeping you full, curbing cravings, and maintaining healthy blood sugar levels. All improve your chances of losing weight.

Plant-Powered Protein Soup

Makes 6 servings

1 tablespoon coconut oil

1 medium onion, chopped

2 cloves garlic, diced

6 cups vegetable stock

1 cup dried yellow split
peas

1 carrot, chopped

3 cups chopped or baby
spinach

1 bay leaf

1 teaspoon sea salt

1 teaspoon ground black
pepper

The right soup can stand on its own as a proper meal. This simple soup is an example. Its split peas pack a serious protein punch. When they're combined with some basic veggies, you've got a quick go-to soup that you can eat fresh and have on hand as leftovers for days. Enjoy this soup on any day other than your Low-Carb Days.

1. In a large pot over medium heat, melt the coconut oil. Add the onion and cook, stirring frequently, for 3 to 4 minutes, or until golden brown.

2. Add the garlic and cook, stirring, for 1 minute. Then add the stock, split peas, carrot, spinach, bay leaf, salt, and pepper. Bring to a boil over medium-high heat, then simmer uncovered for 1 hour.

3. Remove the bay leaf, let the soup cool slightly, then puree it in the pot with an immersion blender or in batches in a blender.

Mighty Minestrone

Makes 6 servings

1 tablespoon coconut oil

1 large onion, chopped

2 cloves garlic, minced

2 large carrots, chopped

6 cups vegetable stock

½ cup quinoa

1 cup canned white beans, rinsed and drained

1 cup kidney beans, rinsed and drained

2 cups chopped green beans

2 large tomatoes, chopped

1 teaspoon dried oregano

1 teaspoon ground black pepper

Minestrone is a thick soup that usually includes pasta or rice. This version, however, is gluten-free and contains only a small amount of quinoa. The rest of the soup's bulk is provided by the protein-, carb-, and fiber-rich white beans and kidney beans. I personally love eating this soup during the cold winter months in Toronto. There's something really soothing about it that just makes you feel good. Enjoy this soup at any time of the year, on any day other than your Low-Carb Days.

1. In a large pot over medium heat, melt the coconut oil. Add the onion and cook, stirring frequently, for 3 minutes, or until softened. Add the garlic and carrots and cook for 1 more minute.

2. Add the stock and bring to a boil, then reduce the heat to simmer. Add the quinoa, beans, and tomatoes and continue to simmer for another 15 minutes.

3. Finish by adding the oregano and pepper. Cook for another 5 minutes. Remove from the heat and let sit for a few minutes before serving.

Zesty Sweet Potato Soup

Makes 4 servings

2 tablespoons coconut oil

1 onion, chopped

2 large sweet potatoes,
   peeled and cubed

1 clove garlic, minced

1 tablespoon curry powder

3 cups vegetable broth

1 cup water

1" piece fresh ginger,
   peeled and grated

Juice of ½ lime

1 cup full-fat canned
   coconut milk

¼ cup chopped fresh
   cilantro

½ teaspoon ground black
   pepper

This is a perfect soup for your 1-Day Feast, as it's loaded with starchy carbs and healthy fats that will keep you full for hours. Remember to watch the calories in recipes like this one, because when you're eating real food, your body will let you know when it's time to stop eating, which is much sooner than if you were eating junk. This soup also provides you with nutrients like ginger and curry powder, which help to keep fat-inducing inflammation in your body at bay.

1. In a medium pot over medium heat, melt the oil. Cook the onion, stirring frequently, for about 2 minutes. Add the sweet potatoes, garlic, and curry and cook, stirring frequently, for 5 minutes, or until the potatoes are slightly softened.

2. Add the broth and water and bring the soup to a boil. Reduce the heat to low and simmer, covered, for 10 minutes or until the potatoes have softened. Add the ginger and let rest for 1 minute.

3. Transfer the soup to a blender, add the lime juice, and blend until smooth. Return it to the pot and keep it on low heat while stirring in the coconut milk, cilantro, and black pepper.

Flavorful Moroccan Chickpea Soup

Feast Approved

Makes 4 servings

2 tablespoons olive oil

3 cloves garlic, minced

1 teaspoon paprika

½ teaspoon ground cumin

½ teaspoon ground
    cinnamon

½ teaspoon coriander
    seeds

2 cups cubed butternut
    squash

1 can (15 ounces)
    chickpeas, rinsed and
    drained

2 large tomatoes, chopped

3 cups vegetable broth

1 tablespoon honey

¼ cup chopped fresh
    cilantro

Juice of ½ lemon

My dad is Moroccan, so I have a natural bias in favor of Moroccan food, which is (in my opinion) the most delicious of all cuisines. It marries spices, herbs, and flavors like no other country's cuisine. This soup is a sampling of the delicious flavors coming out of Morocco. Notice the inclusion of half a dozen herbs and spices in this recipe. After just one spoonful, your taste buds will be begging for more. Enjoy it on any day other than your Low-Carb Days.

1. In a large pot over medium-low heat, place the oil. Add the garlic, paprika, cumin, cinnamon, and coriander seeds and cook, stirring frequently, for 2 minutes. Stir in the squash and chickpeas and cook, stirring occasionally, for another 2 minutes.

2. Add the tomatoes and broth. Increase the heat to high and bring to a boil. Reduce the heat to medium and simmer uncovered for 20 minutes, stirring occasionally.

3. Remove the soup from the heat and stir in the honey, cilantro, and lemon juice. Serve and enjoy.

Creamy Curried Cauliflower Soup

Low Carb

Makes 2 servings

1 tablespoon coconut oil

1 large onion, finely chopped

1 head cauliflower, cut into florets

3 cloves garlic, minced

1 can (14 ounces) full-fat coconut milk

2 cups vegetable stock

½ teaspoon ground coriander

½ teaspoon ground turmeric

½ teaspoon ground cumin

1 teaspoon ground curry powder

¼ cup cashews

Toasted coconut flakes (optional)

Sea salt and ground black pepper

¼ teaspoon ground nutmeg

When I was young, we would have a big Danish smorgasbord (my mom's Danish) every Christmas. Our family friends hosted the festive food onslaught, and it was amazing. One of the wonderful appetizers often served was a cream of cauliflower soup. It was heavy in cream and who knows what else. In an effort to re-create those delicious memories, I came up with this version, adding a hint of curry to make it even more awesome. (If you don't want the curry, then just omit it, along with the turmeric.) You can enjoy this low-carb soup whenever you like.

1. In a large skillet over medium heat, melt the oil. Then add the onion and cauliflower and cook, stirring, for about 1 minute. Turn the heat down to low, cover the pan, and sweat the vegetables for about 10 minutes.

2. Add the garlic, coconut milk, and stock. Turn up the heat until the soup just starts to simmer (do not boil), then put the lid on and turn the heat to low (the soup should still be simmering). Add the coriander, turmeric, cumin, and curry powder and simmer for 10 to 15 minutes. Set aside.

3. Once slightly cooled, carefully add the warm soup to a blender and blend until smooth. Or use an immersion blender right in the pot. Meanwhile, in a small pan over medium heat, toast the cashews for 5 minutes or until lightly brown, stirring frequently.

4. Serve the soup in small bowls, topping it with the cashews and toasted coconut (if using). Add salt and pepper to taste, along with the nutmeg. Enjoy.

Spicy Pea Soup with Swiss Chard

Makes 4 servings

2 tablespoons coconut oil

1 onion, diced

1" piece fresh ginger, peeled and grated

4 cloves garlic, minced

¼ habanero or jalapeño chile pepper, seeded and minced (wear plastic gloves when handling)

1 teaspoon sea salt

Ground black pepper

2 tomatoes, diced

1 teaspoon ground turmeric

1 cup vegetable stock

1 cup full-fat coconut milk

1 can (15 ounces) black-eyed peas, rinsed and drained

4 leaves Swiss chard, stemmed and chopped

1 small handful fresh cilantro, chopped

A little spice is good for you. In fact, most "spicy" spices have a slight metabolism-boosting effect. Now, don't get ahead of yourself and think that by only eating spicy food you're going to turn into a 24/7 fat-burning machine, but every little bit helps. Most spices that pack heat also have very potent anti-inflammatory benefits. So embrace the spice to whatever level you can tolerate. Enjoy this soup on any day other than your Low-Carb Days.

1. In a large pot over medium heat, melt the coconut oil. Cook the onion, stirring frequently, for 3 minutes, or until softened. Add the ginger, garlic, chile pepper, salt, and ground black pepper to taste and cook, stirring occasionally, until softened, about 5 minutes.

2. Add the tomatoes, turmeric, stock, and coconut milk. Bring to a boil, then simmer uncovered over low heat, stirring occasionally, until the tomatoes break down and the sauce thickens a bit, about 20 minutes. Add the peas and Swiss chard and cook over medium-low heat until the peas are lightly coated and the greens are wilted, about 10 minutes. Remove from the heat, stir in the cilantro, and serve.

Sausage, Tomato, and Kale Soup

Makes 4 servings

1 tablespoon coconut oil

4 sausages, sliced (mild
Italian sausage works
well)

½ white onion, diced

2 small cloves garlic,
minced

2 large carrots, chopped

3 scallions, chopped

1 large can (14.5 ounces)
diced tomatoes

4 cups vegetable broth

2 teaspoons dried oregano

1 teaspoon dried basil

3 cups chopped kale, ribs
removed

½ handful parsley,
chopped

Salt and ground black
pepper

Looking for the perfect soup for your Low-Carb Days? Try this one. It provides a healthy dose of protein and overall good nutrition that can be enjoyed whenever you like. This can stand on its own or work as a side or starter alongside any of your favorite mains.

1. In a large pot over medium heat, melt the coconut oil. Add the sausage slices. Cook, stirring, until slightly brown, about 5 minutes. Add the onion, garlic, and carrots and cook, stirring frequently, for about 2 minutes, or until fragrant and soft. Make sure to stir everything around to prevent the garlic and onion from overcooking.

2. Add the scallions and tomatoes. Pour the vegetable broth into the pot and add the oregano and basil. Bring the soup to a boil, then reduce the heat to medium-low and simmer. Toss in the chopped kale and cook for about 5 minutes. Add the parsley, stir, season with salt and pepper to taste, and serve.

No-Cook Ginger Thai Soup

Makes 2 servings

2 carrots

1 red bell pepper

1 can (14 ounces) full-fat
coconut milk

Juice of 1 lime

1" piece fresh ginger,
peeled

2 tablespoons coconut
aminos

1 tablespoon tahini

½ tablespoon maple syrup

2 tablespoons pumpkin
seeds or sunflower
seeds

¼ cup chopped fresh basil

When I was in my midtwenties, I went raw vegan for half a year. I felt amazing, and it really helped turn my health around for the better. Although I don't believe everyone should eat 100 percent raw, I do believe that eating more plant foods in their raw state is the fastest way to have more energy and dramatically improve your health. This soup will give you a feel for what I mean. There's no cooking or heating involved. Simply blend everything together and you're all set—perfect for any day, especially during the warm summer months when you just want something cool and fresh.

In a high-speed blender, combine the carrots, pepper, coconut milk, lime juice, ginger, coconut aminos, tahini, and maple syrup. Puree, adding water if desired, for 20 seconds, or until your preferred consistency is achieved. Top with the pumpkin or sunflower seeds and chopped basil. Serve and enjoy!

Healthy Cream of Mushroom Soup

Makes 4 servings

2 tablespoons coconut oil

1 leek, white and light green parts only, sliced

2 cloves garlic, minced

1 cup chopped shiitake mushrooms

1 cup chopped portobello mushrooms

1 cup chopped cremini mushrooms

¼ cup gluten-free all-purpose flour

1 tablespoon dried thyme

4 cups vegetable broth

1 can (14 ounces) full-fat coconut milk

Sea salt and ground black pepper

My mom used to make mushroom soup all the time when I was growing up. However, it was always from a can and loaded with sodium, dairy, and other nasty ingredients. You know the ones I'm talking about. By contrast, this cream of mushroom soup can be made from scratch in no time. Mushrooms are famous for supporting your immune system, so serve this during cold and flu season, or whenever you feel run-down.

1. In a large pot over medium heat, melt the coconut oil. Add the leek and cook, stirring frequently, for 5 minutes. Add the garlic and cook, stirring frequently, until softened, about 2 minutes.

2. Add the mushrooms and cook for another 10 minutes, or until browned. Add the flour and stir well to combine. Cook for 1 minute longer.

3. Add the thyme, vegetable broth, coconut milk, and salt and pepper to taste. Cook for 15 more minutes.

Bacon-Tomato Zucchini Pasta
(page 185)

Pan-Seared Salmon with Sugar Snap Peas
and Avocado Salad (page 188)

Chicken and Apricot Tagine with
Saffron Quinoa (page 189)

Lemon-Oregano Shrimp with Tomato, Cucumber, and Olive Salad (page 192)

Steak Frites
(page 193)

Curried Chickpea Salad
(page 152)

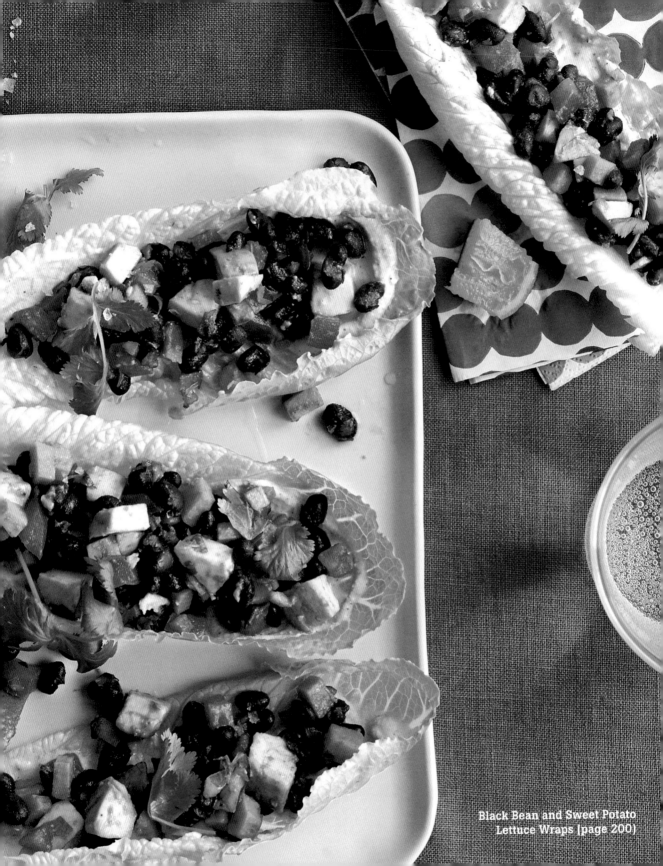

Black Bean and Sweet Potato
Lettuce Wraps (page 200)

Italian Sausage and Roasted
Root Vegetables (page 205)

Set-It-and-Forget-It
Veggie Chili (page 206)

Spicy Greeny Rotini
(page 195)

Peanut Butter Chocolate Balls
(page 211)

Chocolate Chip Oatmeal Cookies
(page 219)

Salted Peanut Butter–Chocolate Pudding
with Coconut Whipped Cream (page 213)

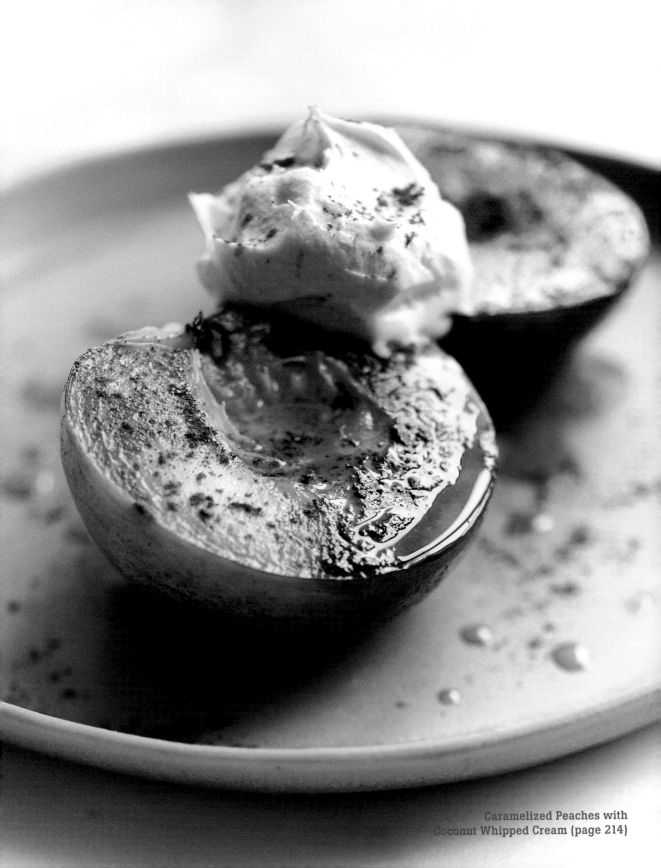

Caramelized Peaches with
Coconut Whipped Cream (page 214)

Apple-Strawberry Crumble
(page 216)

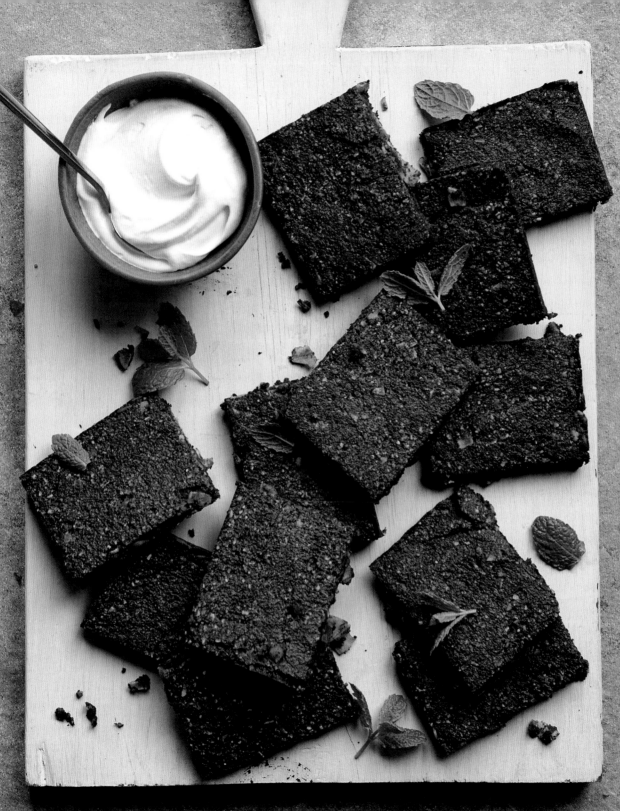

Coco-Chocolate Brownies
(page 218)

Flourless Orange-Almond Cake
(page 215)

Hearty White Bean Soup

Feast Approved

Makes 4 servings

2 tablespoons coconut oil

1 small onion, finely chopped

2 ribs celery, diced

4 cloves garlic, minced

2 teaspoons dried oregano

1 teaspoon dried thyme

1 teaspoon dried basil

2 carrots, diced

2 tomatoes, seeded and chopped

5 cups vegetable stock

2 cans (15 ounces each) cannellini beans, rinsed and drained

10 kale leaves, ribs and stems removed, chopped

Sea salt and ground black pepper

White beans are loaded with antioxidants and provide a good supply of the detoxifying mineral molybdenum. They are also a good source of fiber and protein and are low on the glycemic index, which is good for your blood sugar. Plus they produce alpha-amylase inhibitors, which help regulate fat storage in the body. Think about all that as you enjoy each spoonful of this yummy and hearty soup.

1. Melt the coconut oil in a large pot over medium-high heat. Add the onion, celery, and garlic. Cook for 2 minutes, or until the onions turn translucent. Add the oregano, thyme, basil, carrots, and tomatoes and stir to combine. Cook for about 5 minutes, stirring occasionally.

2. Add the vegetable stock and cannellini beans and bring the soup to a simmer. Simmer it for about 10 minutes, stirring occasionally.

3. Place half of the soup in a blender and blend for 20 seconds, or until creamy. Return it to the pot and stir well to incorporate it. Add the kale and simmer for another 10 minutes. Taste, and add salt and pepper as necessary. Ladle the soup into bowls and enjoy!

Spicy Black Bean Soup

Makes 4 servings

2 tablespoons coconut oil

1 green bell pepper, chopped

2 cloves garlic, chopped

1 large red onion, chopped

1 teaspoon ground cumin

Sea salt and ground black pepper

2 cans (15.5 ounces each) black beans, rinsed and drained

1 cup vegetable broth

3 cups water

1 jalapeño chile pepper, seeded, halved, and chopped (wear plastic gloves when handling)

½ cup chopped fresh cilantro

1 avocado, cubed

Juice of ½ lime

2 tablespoons olive oil

Of all the foods we have access to, no food group has a more health-supportive mix of protein and fiber than legumes, which includes black beans. From a single, 1-cup serving of black beans you get nearly 15 grams of fiber (well over half of the Daily Value) and 15 grams of protein. As such, you can consider this soup a true health tonic that is good for your heart, waistline, gut, and so much more. Enjoy it on any day other than your Low-Carb Days.

1. In a large pot over medium heat, melt the coconut oil. Add the green pepper, garlic, and onion. Cook, stirring occasionally, until tender, about 5 minutes. Stir in the cumin and salt and ground black pepper to taste.

2. Add the beans, broth, and water. Mash some of the beans with a fork. Bring to a boil. Reduce the heat and simmer, stirring occasionally, until the soup is slightly thickened, about 15 minutes.

3. Meanwhile, in a small bowl, toss the chile pepper with the cilantro, avocado, lime juice, olive oil, and additional salt and pepper to taste. Serve on top of the soup.

French Onion Slow-Cooker Soup

Makes 6 servings

2 large sweet onions, sliced

6 cups vegetable or bone broth

Salt and ground black pepper

Chopped parsley, basil, or scallions for garnish (optional)

This slow-cooker soup is good for so many health reasons. On top of that, there's really nothing like enjoying a deeply satisfying, tasty, steaming bowl of this 44-calorie French onion soup.

In a slow cooker, combine the onions and broth. Cover and cook on low for 6 to 8 hours, or on high for 4 to 6 hours. Add salt and pepper to taste. Just before serving, ladle the soup into bowls and garnish with parsley, basil, or scallions, if desired.

Chapter 11

Mains

MOST PEOPLE EAT BECAUSE THEY ARE HUNGRY. My goal is to create healthy meals so good they make you *stop* eating—out of sheer amazement. I believe many of the mains in this section accomplish this goal. Whether you're looking for meat-based or vegan dishes, I have you covered. In each case, you'll experience an explosion of flavors thanks to well-designed herb and spice combinations that will light up your taste buds. Plus all of these meals take less than 20 minutes to prepare. Some require additional cooking time, but your hands-on work will be 20 minutes or less. As a result, you'll look forward to cooking food from scratch because of how good it tastes and how simple it is to make. *Bon appétit!*

Beef and Rice with Spice

Makes 4 servings

Rice

1 tablespoon coconut oil

1" piece fresh ginger, peeled and grated

1 onion, diced

Pinch of sea salt and ground black pepper

1 cup basmati rice

1½ cups water

Spiced Beef

1 tablespoon coconut oil

1 pound ground beef

2 cloves garlic, minced

1 teaspoon ground cumin

1 teaspoon curry powder

Pinch of sea salt and ground black pepper

3 handfuls baby spinach

Juice of ½ lemon

¼ cup chopped almonds, toasted

This simple dish adds flavor and spice to an otherwise boring combination. It's super easy to make and perfect for any day other than your Low-Carb Days. Serve alongside a salad and enjoy.

1. *To make the rice:* In a medium saucepan over medium heat, melt the coconut oil. Cook the ginger, onion, and salt and pepper for about 5 minutes. Stir in the rice and cook, stirring, until lightly toasted, about 3 minutes.

2. Stir in the water and bring to a boil. Reduce the heat, cover, and simmer until no liquid remains, about 15 minutes. Then remove from the heat.

3. *To make the beef:* At the same, in a large skillet over medium heat, melt the coconut oil. Add the ground beef and cook for about 2 minutes. Stir in the garlic, cumin, curry powder, and salt and pepper. Continue cooking and stirring until the beef is no longer pink, about 5 minutes. Stir in the spinach, lemon juice, and chopped almonds.

4. Combine the beef mixture and the rice, serve, and enjoy.

Bacon-Tomato Zucchini Pasta

Makes 2 servings

1 cup cherry tomatoes

1 teaspoon sea salt

1 teaspoon ground black pepper

2 strips bacon

1 teaspoon minced garlic

1 teaspoon red-pepper flakes

3 cups baby spinach or chopped spinach

1 large zucchini, peeled

1 tablespoon olive oil

You don't need traditional grain-based pastas when you can use good old zucchini. This aromatic, light pasta is brought to life even further with the addition of bacon. If you want to keep it vegan, then omit the bacon. If you need a little more substance to your meal, then pair this with one of the sides or salads from an earlier chapter.

1. Preheat the oven to 400°F. Place the tomatoes on a baking sheet and season with the salt and pepper. Bake for 15 minutes. Set aside.

2. Meanwhile, place a large skillet over medium heat. Cook the bacon for 3 minutes, then flip it over and cook for another 3 to 5 minutes or to your preferred crispiness. Place the bacon on a plate covered with paper towels to absorb the excess fat.

3. Pour half of the bacon fat out of the skillet. Cook the garlic for 1 minute, then add the red-pepper flakes and spinach. Cook for 5 minutes, or until the spinach is mostly wilted. At the same time, run the zucchini through a spiralizer to create spaghetti-like noodles (or use a vegetable peeler to slice fettuccine-like noodles if you don't have a spiralizer).

4. Add the zucchini, roasted tomatoes, and bacon to the skillet. Stir frequently for 1 to 2 minutes, or until the noodles are coated with the tomato juices and have softened. Drizzle with the olive oil and enjoy.

Zucchini Pesto Pasta with Sliced Chicken

Low Carb

Makes 2 servings

Pesto

1 clove garlic

1 cup fresh basil

¾ cup pine nuts

3 tablespoons olive oil

1 teaspoon sea salt

1 tablespoon lemon juice

Zucchini Pasta

1 tablespoon coconut oil

1 medium chicken breast, halved and sliced into strips

1 teaspoon salt

1 teaspoon ground black pepper

1 large zucchini, peeled

1 cup halved cherry tomatoes

This zucchini pasta is served raw and topped with sautéed chicken. You can omit the chicken if you want to keep it vegan. Otherwise, the chicken is a really nice complement to the pesto sauce. This is a great low-carb dish to enjoy on any day when you want pasta but without the carbs of traditional noodles.

---

1. *To make the pesto:* In a food processor, combine the garlic, basil, pine nuts, olive oil, sea salt, and lemon juice. Process until creamy.

2. *To make the pasta:* In a medium skillet over medium heat, melt the coconut oil. Add the chicken strips. Season with the salt and pepper and cook, turning frequently, for 3 to 5 minutes, or until the chicken is no longer pink.

3. At the same time, use a julienne peeler or spiralizer to slice the zucchini into noodles. Place the noodles in a large serving bowl, along with the tomatoes and pesto. Top with the chicken, toss well, and serve.

Sinfully Good Shrimp Penne

Makes 4 servings

1 pound gluten-free penne

2 tablespoons butter

4 cloves garlic, minced

½ teaspoon fennel seeds

½ teaspoon hot-pepper
flakes

1 pound medium shrimp,
peeled and deveined

3 large tomatoes, chopped

¼ cup chopped parsley

2 tablespoons capers

Juice of ½ lemon

1 teaspoon sea salt

This recipe calls for any type of gluten-free penne noodles and is a little more carb heavy than its zucchini pasta predecessors. When combined with shrimp and some great herbs and spices, you've got a simple dish we often make at home when our kids are begging for pasta. It's healthy and keeps them happy—so everyone wins.

1. Cook the penne according to package instructions until al dente. Drain, reserving 2 tablespoons of the liquid.

2. Meanwhile, in a large skillet over medium heat, melt the butter. Cook the garlic, fennel seeds, hot-pepper flakes, and shrimp, stirring frequently, for 2 minutes. Stir in the tomatoes and cook for 5 minutes longer, or until the shrimp is pink.

3. Add the parsley, capers, lemon juice, the reserved pasta-cooking liquid, and salt and cook, stirring frequently, for 1 minute. Finish by combining the pasta with the shrimp mixture in the skillet. Mix well and serve.

Pan–Seared Salmon with Sugar Snap Peas and Avocado Salad

Makes 3 to 4 servings

2 salmon fillets (about 6 ounces each)

1 teaspoon sea salt

½ teaspoon ground black pepper

2 tablespoons coconut oil

4 cups sugar snap peas, trimmed

1 tablespoon apple cider vinegar

2 tablespoons olive oil

1 teaspoon coconut aminos or tamari

1 teaspoon Dijon mustard

½ teaspoon sesame oil

1 clove garlic, crushed and minced

1 tablespoon sesame seeds, lightly toasted

4 scallions, sliced

1 avocado, cubed

Salmon pairs really well with a variety of vegetables. Here, we're tossing together a fresh snap pea and avocado salad with a lovely vinaigrette and having that alongside the salmon. This is another easy dinner to whip together if you're pressed for time and is perfect for any day other than your Low-Carb Days.

1. Season both sides of the salmon with the sea salt and pepper and let rest for a moment. Meanwhile, in a medium pan over medium-low heat, melt the coconut oil. Cook the salmon for 6 to 8 minutes, turning once, or until opaque, being careful not to burn either side.

2. At the same time, add the snap peas to a large pot of boiling salted water. Cook for 2 minutes, drain, and transfer to a bowl of ice water to chill. Drain well and set aside.

3. Meanwhile, in a large bowl, whisk together the vinegar, olive oil, coconut aminos or tamari, mustard, sesame oil, and garlic until well combined. Stir in the sesame seeds and scallions. Then stir in the sugar snap peas and avocado, toss to combine, and serve alongside the salmon.

Chicken and Apricot Tagine
with Saffron Quinoa

Makes 4 servings

2 tablespoons coconut oil

2 onions, minced

4 cloves garlic, minced

2 bone-in chicken breasts

2 bone-in chicken legs

1 can (28 ounces) diced
tomatoes, undrained

½ teaspoon ground
cinnamon

½" piece fresh ginger,
peeled and grated

½ teaspoon ground black
pepper

1 teaspoon ground cumin

1 teaspoon coriander
seeds

1 teaspoon sea salt

1 cup dried apricots

½ cup chopped fresh
cilantro

1½ cups quinoa

3 cups water

1 teaspoon saffron

This is one of the tastiest dishes in this entire cookbook. I bet it will even become one of your all-time favorites if you enjoy the combination of apricot and a host of savory spices. To make this taste even better, let the chicken sit in the apricot tagine for as long as you can. Doing so will make the chicken fall-off-the-bone tender. To get the most from each bite, take a forkful of chicken, apricot, and saffron quinoa—the flavors are seriously amazing when eaten together.

Saffron isn't the most common spice, so if you can find it, great! Please use it here. If not, don't worry about it— this dish will still taste great.

1. In a large pot over medium heat, melt the coconut oil. Cook the onions and garlic, stirring frequently, for 1 minute. Add the chicken and cook until lightly browned, about 5 minutes, turning occasionally.

2. Add the tomatoes, cinnamon, ginger, pepper, cumin, coriander seeds, and salt. Bring to a boil, then reduce the heat and simmer, covered, for 1 hour. Add the apricots and simmer for another hour. During the last few minutes of that hour, add the cilantro.

3. Meanwhile, in a medium pot, combine the quinoa and water. Bring to a boil over high heat. Cover, reduce the heat to low, and simmer until the quinoa is tender, about 15 minutes. Add the saffron about halfway through the cooking process.

4. To serve, place the quinoa on a large serving platter, then top it with the chicken tagine mixture.

Fast and Flavorful Chicken and Veggies

Makes 2 servings

1 quart chicken or
   vegetable broth

3 cloves garlic, minced

2 sprigs fresh thyme

1 bay leaf

1 bulb fennel, chopped

2 cups halved Brussels
   sprouts

2 medium carrots,
   chopped into 1" pieces

2 scallions, chopped

2 boneless, skinless
   chicken breasts, sliced

If you just want to whip together some chicken and veggies, then go with this simple recipe. There's nothing fancy about, and it will serve well on both Low-Carb Days and Low-Cal Days. It's light, fresh, and any leftovers can be packed up if you need something to take with you to work.

1. In a large pot over high heat, bring the broth, garlic, thyme, and bay leaf to a boil. Add the fennel, Brussels sprouts, and carrots and cook for 10 minutes, or until desired tenderness. Add the scallions and cook for 1 minute. Using a slotted spoon, remove the vegetables, place them in a large bowl, and cover it with foil.

2. Add the chicken to the pot and cook for 3 minutes. Cover and remove from the heat. Let stand until the chicken is cooked through, about 15 minutes. Remove the chicken with the slotted spoon, plate it alongside the vegetables, and moisten everything by adding a splash of broth.

Sweet-and-Sour Sautéed Salmon with Baby Bok Choy

Low Carb

Makes 2 servings

Salmon

1 tablespoon maple syrup

1 tablespoon coconut aminos or tamari

1 red chile pepper, seeded and minced

2 cloves garlic, minced

2 tablespoons chopped shallots

1 teaspoon sea salt

½ teaspoon ground pepper

2 salmon fillets (about 6 ounces each)

1 tablespoon coconut oil

¼ cup chopped fresh cilantro

Juice of ½ lemon

Bok Choy

10 baby bok choy, trimmed

2 tablespoons coconut oil

2 cloves garlic, minced

Juice of ½ lemon

2 teaspoons grated lemon peel

½ teaspoon sea salt

¼ teaspoon ground pepper

There are many ways to prepare salmon. This dish features the contrasting flavors of maple syrup and coconut aminos or tamari, which taste a bit like soy sauce. The result is a sweet-and-sour combo that coats the salmon perfectly. Although there's a smidgen of maple syrup here, I still consider this recipe okay for a Low-Carb Day.

1. *To make the salmon:* In a large bowl, combine the maple syrup, coconut aminos or tamari, chile pepper (wear plastic gloves), garlic, shallots, salt, and black pepper. Place the salmon in the bowl, cover with plastic wrap, and marinate for 30 minutes.

2. In a large skillet over medium heat, melt the coconut oil. Add the salmon, along with the marinade, and cook for 6 to 8 minutes, turning at least once, or until the salmon is opaque and lightly caramelized. Put the salmon on a serving plate. Pour the remaining marinade over it and top with the cilantro. Drizzle with the lemon juice. Keep warm.

3. *To make the bok choy:* Meanwhile, in a steamer over high heat, cook the bok choy for 4 to 5 minutes. Remove the steamer from the heat and keep it covered.

4. Melt the coconut oil in a large skillet over medium heat. Cook the garlic, lemon juice, and lemon peel, stirring frequently, for 30 seconds. Add the bok choy, salt, and pepper and cook for 2 to 3 minutes longer. Once the desired tenderness is achieved, remove the bok choy from the skillet and serve it alongside the salmon.

Lemon–Oregano Shrimp with Tomato, Cucumber, and Olive Salad

Low Carb

Makes 4 servings

Salad

½ **medium cucumber, thinly sliced**

2 **cups halved cherry tomatoes**

1 **cup pitted and halved kalamata olives**

2 **tablespoons olive oil**

1 **tablespoon lemon juice**

½ **teaspoon dried oregano**

½ **teaspoon dried thyme**

Shrimp

2 **tablespoons butter**

3 **cloves garlic, minced**

1 **tablespoon chopped fresh oregano or 1 teaspoon dried**

1 **pound fresh or frozen and thawed large shrimp, peeled and deveined**

1 **teaspoon sea salt**

Juice of ½ lemon

Shrimp is a really good source of protein. It's also very versatile, lending itself to countless flavor and food-pairing combinations. In this recipe, you'll enjoy a whirlwind of flavors, since everything is tossed together in a salad—perfect to enjoy fresh or to take with you when you're on the go. This is a low-carb dish that can be enjoyed anytime. Pair it with your favorite side if you need some more substance.

1. *To make the salad:* In a large bowl, combine the cucumber, tomatoes, olives, olive oil, lemon juice, oregano, and thyme. Toss well.

2. *To make the shrimp:* In a large skillet over medium heat, melt the butter. Cook the garlic, stirring frequently, for 2 minutes, then add the oregano. Add the shrimp and cook, stirring occasionally, until the shrimp turn pink, about 4 minutes. Sprinkle in the salt and lemon juice and cook for 1 more minute, then remove from the heat. Toss together with the salad and serve.

Olive Oil Facilitates Fat Loss

Numerous studies have linked Mediterranean dietary patterns, rich in olive oil, with favorable effects on body weight. In one 2½-year study of more than 7,000 Spanish college students, consuming a lot of olive oil was not linked to increased weight.[1] And another 3-year study found that a diet rich in olive oil increased levels of antioxidants in the blood and facilitated weight loss.[2]

Steak Frites

1 pound yellow potatoes, quartered into wedges

3 tablespoons melted butter, divided

12 ounces sirloin steak

3 sprigs fresh thyme

1 teaspoon sea salt

½ teaspoon ground black pepper

1 tablespoon chopped fresh chives

2 teaspoons Dijon mustard

⅓ cup Metabolic Mayo (page 131)

Juice of ½ lemon

Yes, indeed! That's what we're doing here—the classic steak frites. How this dish turns out is entirely dependent on the quality of the steak you choose and how you cook it. I like my steak medium-rare, but whatever works best for you is all that matters. Instead of relying on potatoes fried in oil (aka French fries), we're going to roast ours in the oven. Feel free to cut the potatoes into frylike sticks instead of wedges, if you prefer. As there are no veggies in this dish, choose a salad to go alongside it. You can enjoy this dish on any day other than your Low-Carb Days.

1. Preheat the oven to 450°F and line a baking sheet with parchment paper.

2. In a large bowl, toss the potatoes with 2 tablespoons of the butter. Spread the potatoes on the baking sheet and bake until tender, about 15 minutes, turning once. Then broil the potatoes until golden brown, about 2 minutes.

3. Meanwhile, sprinkle the steak with the thyme, salt, and pepper. In a large skillet over medium-high heat, cook the steak in the remaining 1 tablespoon melted butter, turning once, for 2 to 3 minutes per side, or until a thermometer inserted in the center registers 145°F for medium-rare/160°F for medium/165°F for well-done. Transfer the steak to a cutting board, tent with foil, and let stand for 10 minutes.

4. In a small bowl, stir together the chives, mustard, Metabolic Mayo, and lemon juice. Serve with the steak, as a dipping sauce for the frites.

Finger-Lickin' Chicken Salad

Makes 2 servings

2 chicken breasts, halved, then cut into strips

1 teaspoon sea salt

½ teaspoon ground black pepper

1 tablespoon coconut oil

1 tablespoon sesame seeds

Juice of ½ lime

1" piece fresh ginger, peeled and grated

1 teaspoon honey

2 tablespoons olive oil

1 tablespoon apple cider vinegar

1 tablespoon Dijon mustard

1 clove garlic, minced

½ bulb fennel, cored and thinly sliced

2 cups shredded red cabbage

1 orange, peeled and quartered

½ cup chopped fresh cilantro

Chicken works really well with oranges. And oranges go really well with fennel. In this salad, we're going to throw them all together, along with shredded cabbage and a flavor-packed dressing. With meals like this, chicken doesn't have to be dry and boring. Enjoy on any day other than your Low-Carb Days.

1. Season the chicken with the salt and pepper. In a medium skillet over medium heat, melt the coconut oil. Cook the chicken until no longer pink and the juices run clear, about 5 minutes.

2. Meanwhile, in a small bowl, stir together the sesame seeds, lime juice, ginger, and honey. Pour the mixture over the chicken and cook for 1 minute longer.

3. In a large bowl, combine the olive oil, vinegar, mustard, and garlic. Add the fennel, red cabbage, orange, and cilantro. Then add the chicken, toss well, and serve.

Spicy Greeny Rotini

Makes 4 servings

6 cups gluten-free rotini

1 bunch asparagus, thick stalks removed, cut into 1" pieces

2 cups broccolini florets

2 tablespoons olive oil

4 cloves garlic, minced

1 teaspoon red-pepper flakes

1 teaspoon dried oregano

2 chorizo sausages or Italian sausages, sliced

Juice of ½ lemon

1 teaspoon sea salt

½ teaspoon ground black pepper

In the mood for a comforting pasta? If so, you're in luck. This is another favorite in my house. Since kids generally love pasta, it's pretty easy to sneak in some other delicious ingredients (including veggies) and allow the pasta to shuttle them into their little bodies. This is also a great meal for after a workout, when your muscles are most receptive to carb intake. Enjoy on any day other than your Low-Carb Days.

1. Cook the rotini according to package instructions, adding the asparagus and broccolini during the last 3 minutes of cooking. Drain, reserving ½ cup of the pasta-cooking liquid.

2. Meanwhile, in a large skillet over medium-low heat, heat the oil. Cook the garlic, red-pepper flakes, and oregano, stirring, until the garlic is golden, about 2 minutes. Add the sausage and cook until lightly browned, about 5 minutes.

3. Stir in the pasta, asparagus, broccolini, reserved pasta-cooking liquid, lemon juice, salt, and black pepper. Cook, stirring, for 1 minute, then remove from the heat and serve.

Chicken and Vegetable Curry

Makes 4 servings

1 tablespoon coconut oil

1 medium onion, chopped

1 medium carrot, diced

4 boneless, skinless
    chicken thighs, cut into
    1" pieces

4 cloves garlic, crushed

3 tablespoons curry paste

1 teaspoon garam masala

1 head broccoli, broken
    into small florets

1 handful green beans,
    trimmed

1 can (14 ounces) full-fat
    coconut milk

1 tablespoon coconut
    sugar or brown sugar

1 teaspoon sea salt

Ground black pepper

½ handful fresh cilantro,
    chopped

Indian food is one of my favorite cuisines. It's all about the spices, really. This dish will give you a sense of what I mean, with an array of different flavors that blend together in a coconut-based curry that takes regular chicken to the next level. Plus curry is a great anti-inflammatory spice, which is great for our goal of burning fat. This low-carb dish is perfect for any day and lends itself nicely to leftovers. Serve with Cauliflower Rice (page 114) if you want to add a little more substance to the dish while keeping it a low-carb meal.

1. In a large skillet over medium-high heat, melt the coconut oil. Cook the onion and carrot, stirring frequently, for 3 minutes, or until the onion becomes soft and transparent. Add the chicken and cook for 5 minutes, or until no longer pink. Add the garlic, curry paste, and garam masala, and cook, stirring together to blend, for about 1 minute.

2. Add the broccoli florets and green beans and continue cooking while stirring occasionally for 5 minutes. Add the coconut milk and sugar, stir well, and bring to a simmer. Reduce the heat to low, add the salt and pepper to taste, and continue to simmer for 10 to 15 minutes, or until the broccoli has reached the desired softness. Garnish with the cilantro before serving.

Tasty Thai Stir-Fry

Makes 2 to 3 servings

Thai Sauce

¼ cup sesame oil

2" piece fresh ginger,
  peeled and grated

8 cloves garlic, minced

½ cup raw sunflower seeds

1 cup unsweetened dried
  coconut

2 tablespoons chili powder

Juice of 1 lemon

2 tablespoons coconut
  aminos

3 cups carrot juice

1 teaspoon paprika

Pinch of sea salt

Ground black pepper

Noodles

3 cups rice noodles

3 handfuls chopped
  greens (bok choy, kale)

1 tomato, chopped

1 handful fresh bean sprouts

Juice of ½ lime

1 small handful cilantro,
  chopped

½ cup chopped peanuts
  (optional)

Stir-fries are all about the sauce, if you ask me. Sure, you can sauté a bunch of veggies, but it's the sauce that brings it all together and makes you beg for more. If you like Thai food, then you'll love the Thai sauce that goes into this stir-fry. It's simply awesome! Enjoy this dish on any day other than your Low-Carb Days.

1. *To make the sauce:* In a large skillet over medium heat, warm the sesame oil. Add the ginger and garlic and cook, stirring frequently, for about 5 minutes. Meanwhile, in a food processor (or blender or coffee grinder), grind the sunflower seeds to a coarse meal.

2. Add the ground sunflower seeds, coconut, chili powder, lemon juice, coconut aminos, carrot juice, paprika, salt, and pepper to taste to the skillet and stir well to combine. Bring the mixture to a boil and then simmer for 15 minutes.

3. *To make the noodles:* While the sauce is cooking, soak the noodles in warm water for about 15 minutes. Place in a colander to drain.

4. In a wok over medium heat, combine the greens, tomato, and Thai sauce. Bring to a boil, then reduce the heat and simmer for 5 minutes. Toss the soaked noodles into the wok and continue to simmer until the noodles are soft, about 2 minutes.

5. Remove from the heat and garnish with the bean sprouts, lime juice, cilantro, and chopped peanuts (if desired).

Baked Citrus Fillet of Sole

Makes 2 servings

1 cup cherry tomatoes

½ bulb fennel, sliced

2 tablespoons coconut oil
   or butter

Sea salt and ground black
   pepper

2 sole fillets (4 to 6 ounces
   each)

1 lemon, quartered

2 sprigs fresh tarragon

Sole is a very light fish. It's a nice change from salmon, which is quite a bit heavier. This low-carb dish is great for your Low-Cal Days and Low-Carb Days. Pair it with a nice salad or side, and you're all set. Don't forget to drizzle lemon juice over the top of the sole before serving to make it taste even better.

1. Preheat the oven to 375°F. In an ovenproof 13" x 9" baking dish, toss the tomatoes and fennel with the oil or butter. Sprinkle with salt and pepper to taste and bake for 15 minutes, or until tender.

2. Add the sole fillets, lemon quarters, and tarragon to the dish, cover with a lid or foil, and bake for another 10 to 12 minutes, or until the sole is cooked through but not dry. Squeeze the lemon quarters over the sole and serve it alongside your favorite salad.

Salmon, Asparagus, Avocado, and Dill Salad

Low Carb

Makes 2 servings

1 tablespoon butter

1 salmon fillet (6 ounces)

8 spears asparagus, trimmed

1 handful salad greens

1 tablespoon capers

1 avocado, cubed

3 tablespoons chopped fresh dill

Juice of ½ lemon

2 tablespoons olive oil

Sea salt and ground black pepper

This is a fun meal because you're taking three foods that could sit beside each other on a plate and, instead, tossing them together in a colorful and flavorful salad. It's a quick dinner option, and you can take any leftovers with you the next day if you're on the go.

1. In a large skillet over medium heat, melt the butter. Cook the salmon for 6 to 8 minutes, turning once, or until the salmon is opaque but has a hint of pink still remaining inside. Remove from the heat and set aside to cool slightly, then cut into bite-size portions.

2. Meanwhile, in a steamer, cook the asparagus for 5 minutes, or until the desired softness is achieved. (Alternatively, you can enjoy the asparagus raw.) Chop into 1"-long pieces.

3. In a large bowl, combine the salad greens, capers, asparagus, salmon, avocado, dill, lemon juice, olive oil, and salt and pepper to taste. Toss well and serve.

Black Bean and Sweet Potato Lettuce Wraps

Feast Approved

Makes 12 (4 servings)

1 sweet potato

⅓ cup coconut cream (the solids at the top of a can of coconut milk)

Juice of 1 lime

½ teaspoon chili powder

¼ teaspoon ground cumin

Sea salt

2 tablespoons apple cider vinegar

1 tablespoon coconut oil, melted

1 can (15 ounces) black beans, rinsed and drained

¼ red onion, finely chopped

1 avocado, diced

1 tomato, diced

¼ cup chopped fresh cilantro

Ground black pepper

12 romaine lettuce leaves

This filling, plant-based dinner is full of incredible flavor combos. Sweet potato, black beans, and avocado make a rich and creamy meal. Spiked with a spicy coconut cream, this dinner is a great way to eat plant-based foods without feeling like a rabbit!

1. Preheat the oven to 350°F. Pierce the sweet potato and bake it for 25 to 30 minutes, or until crisp-tender. Remove from the oven to cool, then peel and dice.

2. In a small bowl, stir together the coconut cream, lime juice, chili powder, cumin, and a pinch of salt. Set aside.

3. In a medium bowl, mix together the sweet potatoes, vinegar, coconut oil, black beans, onion, avocado, tomato, and cilantro. Lightly salt and pepper to taste.

4. Spread the coconut cream on the romaine leaves. Top with the sweet potato and black bean mixture. Enjoy taco-style!

Garlic Veggie Kabobs

Makes 8 (2 to 3 servings)

2 cups chopped portobello mushrooms (2" pieces)

Juice of 2 medium limes

4 cloves garlic, minced

3 tablespoons coconut oil, melted

Sea salt and freshly ground black pepper

1 zucchini, sliced into 1" pieces

1 yellow bell pepper, sliced into 2" pieces

1 green bell pepper, sliced into 2" pieces

1 red onion, sliced into eighths

Here's a perfect low-carb vegan option for a barbecue or a nice summer meal outdoors. It's simple to make and packs tons of lovely colors and flavors, which is synonymous with excellent nutrition. You can enjoy these kabobs on their own or alongside any of the sides and salads throughout this cookbook.

1. In a large bowl, combine the mushrooms, lime juice, garlic, coconut oil, and salt and black pepper to taste. Let sit for 20 minutes.

2. Add the zucchini, bell peppers, and red onion and toss well. Thread the veggies and mushrooms onto 8 wooden skewers and set aside. Meanwhile, preheat the grill to medium-high.

3. Brush the grill grate with coconut oil. Place the kabobs directly on the grill and cook for 2 to 3 minutes per side, or until the veggies are soft. Serve over quinoa or alongside your favorite side or salad.

Broccoli-Chicken Skillet

Low Carb

Makes 2 servings

2 tablespoons coconut oil

2 boneless, skinless
   chicken breasts, cubed

Sea salt and freshly
   ground black pepper

1 onion, chopped

3 cloves garlic, minced

2 cups broccoli florets

2 cups chopped fresh
   spinach

2 teaspoons chili powder

½ tablespoon paprika

½ cup chopped almonds

1 large avocado, sliced

This is a convenient one-pan meal. Broccoli contains potent antioxidants and anti-inflammatory compounds, so eating broccoli on a regular basis will greatly benefit your health. And it certainly doesn't hurt to wrap it in delicious flavors like you'll experience in this meal.

1. In a large skillet over medium-high heat, melt the coconut oil. Add the chicken and salt and pepper to taste and cook until no longer pink, 2 to 3 minutes.

2. Add the onion, garlic, broccoli, spinach, chili powder, and paprika and cook, stirring frequently, until soft, about 10 minutes. Serve with the chopped almonds and sliced avocado.

Dill-Roasted Veggies and Salmon

Makes 2 to 3 servings

2 tablespoons butter,
melted

½ cup halved cherry
tomatoes

½ large yellow squash,
chopped

¼ cup chopped Brussels
sprouts

¼ onion, chopped

1 tablespoon chopped
fresh dill

2 cloves garlic, minced

1 teaspoon chili powder

2 sockeye salmon fillets
(6 ounces each)

Sea salt and freshly
ground black pepper

Dill and salmon go together like soup and salad. In this dish, we're throwing together a bunch of veggies and infusing them with aromatic dill, then topping them off with salmon. It all roasts together in the oven to allow the flavors to work their magic. This is an easy and nutritious meal that's perfect for a hectic weeknight dinner.

1. Preheat the oven to 375°F. In a greased 13" x 9" roasting pan, toss together the butter, tomatoes, squash, Brussels sprouts, onion, dill, garlic, and chili powder. Place the salmon fillets on top of the vegetables and season everything to taste with salt and pepper.

2. Roast in the oven for about 20 minutes, or until the salmon is opaque and the veggies are tender. Remove from the oven and let rest for 3 to 5 minutes before serving.

Honey-Sesame Chicken Stir-Fry

Feast Approved

Makes 2 servings

1 tablespoon coconut oil

2 boneless, skinless
  chicken breasts, sliced

1 onion, diced

2 cloves garlic, minced

1 carrot, cut into coins

1 head broccoli, cut into
  florets

2 tablespoons raw honey

2 tablespoons coconut
  aminos

1 tablespoon sesame
  seeds

Have you ever gone to a Chinese buffet, wound up eating two platefuls too many, and felt like falling asleep soon after? I sure have. This is not only because of the sheer volume of food, but many dishes in these lower-end buffets use terrible ingredients in their sauces, especially monosodium glutamate (MSG), which negatively affects a lot of people. So if you still want to eat yummy Chinese food but in a healthier manner, replace the MSG-loaded Chinese take-out with this homemade sweet and sticky chicken stir-fry. Serve with Cauliflower Rice (page 114) and a salad or a side of greens on any day other than your Low-Carb Days.

1. In a large skillet over medium-high heat, melt the coconut oil. Add the chicken and cook, stirring, for 5 minutes, or until lightly golden and cooked through. Remove from the pan.

2. In the same pan, cook the onion and garlic for 3 minutes, or until the onion starts to soften. Add the carrot and broccoli and cook for 2 to 3 more minutes. Stir the honey and coconut aminos throughout the vegetables. Add the chicken back to the pan and cook until everything is heated through.

3. Divide the stir-fry between 2 plates and sprinkle the sesame seeds on top.

Italian Sausage and Roasted Root Vegetables

Feast Approved

Makes 3 to 4 servings

4 Italian sausages, cut into 1"-thick slices

1 Granny Smith apple, peeled, cored, and cubed

2 cups cubed butternut squash

1 cup halved Brussels sprouts, outer leaves removed

1 red onion, quartered

4 small purple potatoes or 1 sweet potato, cubed

3 cloves garlic, minced

3 tablespoons butter or coconut oil, melted

1 teaspoon dried thyme

1 teaspoon dried rosemary

Sea salt and ground black pepper

If autumn flavors are what you crave, try this warm and comforting roasted root vegetable dish. You'll get a nutritious dinner loaded with apples, butternut squash, and Brussels sprouts. This combination of flavors, along with the saltiness of the sausage, will excite your taste buds. When you've got meals this good and healthy, it's hard not to eat well.

Preheat the oven to 375°F. In a large roasting pan, toss the sausages, apple, squash, Brussels sprouts, red onion, potatoes, and garlic with the butter or coconut oil. Season with the thyme, rosemary, and salt and pepper to taste. Bake for 20 to 25 minutes.

Set-It-and-Forget-It Veggie Chili

Makes 6 servings

1 medium red onion,
  chopped

1 bell pepper (any color),
  seeded and chopped

4 cloves garlic, chopped

1 tablespoon chili powder

1 teaspoon ground cumin

2 teaspoons unsweetened
  cocoa powder

1 teaspoon ground
  cinnamon

1 teaspoon sea salt

½ teaspoon ground black
  pepper

1 can (28 ounces) fire-
  roasted diced tomatoes,
  undrained

1 can (15.5 ounces) kidney
  beans, rinsed and
  drained

1 can (15 ounces) pinto
  beans, rinsed and
  drained

1 medium sweet potato,
  peeled and cut into
  ½" pieces

1 cup vegetable broth

Sliced scallions

Avocado, cubed

I love chili. It's a surefire dish that gives you all the fiber, protein, and healthy carbs you need to keep going for hours. Because of this recipe's inclusion of starchy carbs (in the form of sweet potatoes and beans), this chili is also a perfect meal for your 1-Day Feast or Regular-Cal Days.

This recipe is meant to be prepared in a slow cooker. It requires about 15 minutes of prep work, and then you can let it sit all day (or overnight) to cook and bring all its magical flavors together. If you don't have a slow cooker, you can still simmer this recipe in a large, covered pot on your stove top. Just keep an eye on it and give it the occasional stir.

1. In a slow cooker, combine the onion, bell pepper, garlic, chili powder, cumin, cocoa, cinnamon, salt, and black pepper. Add the tomatoes (and their liquid), beans, sweet potato, and broth.

2. Cover and cook on low until the sweet potatoes are tender and the chili has thickened, 5 to 6 hours. Alternatively, cook the chili on high for 2 to 3 hours. Garnish with the sliced scallions and cubed avocado.

One-Pot Chicken Alfredo

Makes 2 servings

8 ounces gluten-free brown rice pasta

3 cloves garlic, finely chopped

2 tablespoons nutritional yeast

1 chicken breast, cooked and cubed

1 cup coconut milk

2 tablespoons olive oil

2 cups vegetable or chicken broth (high-protein bone broth preferred)

½ teaspoon salt

This rich and creamy, one-pot pasta recipe makes a hearty gluten-free, dairy-free, and stress-free weeknight meal.

1. In a large saucepan, combine the pasta, garlic, yeast, chicken, coconut milk, olive oil, broth, and salt.

2. Cover the saucepan and bring to a boil over medium-high heat.

3. Stir every 2 to 3 minutes to keep the noodles from sticking to each other.

4. Remove from stove once al dente, after 12 to 15 minutes of cooking.

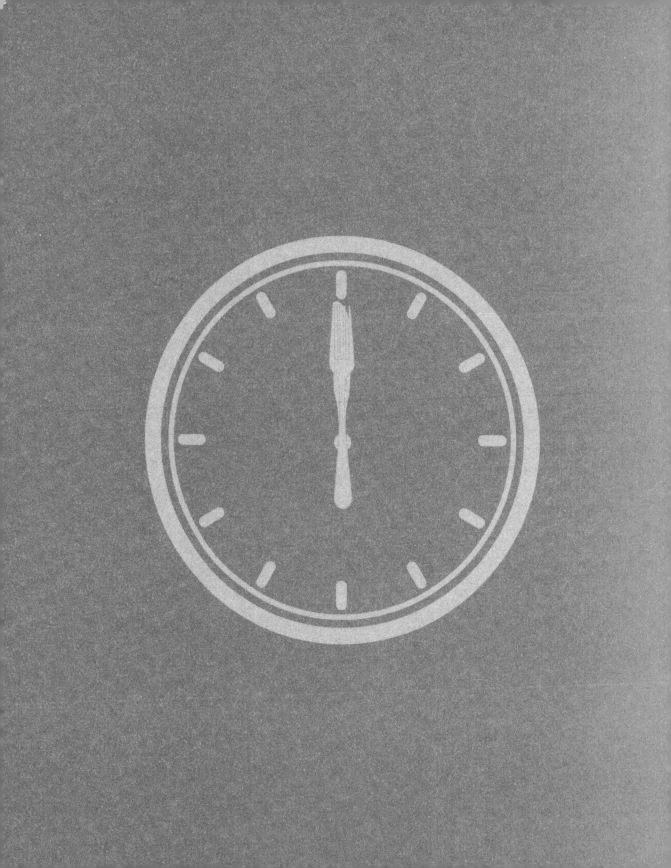

Chapter 12

Desserts

WHO DOESN'T LIKE DESSERT? No matter how much we eat, there always seems to be room for dessert. That's partly because our brain's reward center lights up with dopamine when we eat sweet treats. Unfortunately, most desserts are loaded with sugar, wheat, and dairy—all of which pack on the pounds and leave you feeling out of sorts. By contrast, the recipes in this section are all gluten- and dairy-free and low in sugar. The ones that do contain a little more natural sugar (in the form of fruit) are well balanced with protein and fiber to reduce its impact. In many cases, you can have these desserts as snacks throughout the day—that's how healthy they are. But please remember that the poison is in the dose, so don't go crazy with dessert on a daily basis. Once in a while is fine, especially on your 1-Day Feasts.

Coco-Goji Balls

Makes 10

1½ cups unsweetened
    shredded coconut,
    divided

2 tablespoons hemp seeds

3 tablespoons coconut oil,
    melted

1 tablespoon maple syrup

Juice of ½" piece peeled
    and grated fresh ginger

½ teaspoon vanilla extract

¼ teaspoon sea salt

¼ cup goji berries

Did you know that goji berries are one of the top sources of antioxidants on the planet? Not only that, but they're well known for their polysaccharides, a type of carbohydrate famous for improving communication between immune cells in your body. These balls make a great dessert as well as a healthy on-the-go snack, and they're perfect for a Low-Carb Day.

1. Line a baking sheet with parchment paper. Place ¼ cup of the coconut on a plate.

2. In a food processor, combine the remaining 1¼ cups coconut, hemp seeds, coconut oil, maple syrup, ginger juice, vanilla, and salt. Process until the mixture becomes a thick paste. Add the goji berries and pulse to combine.

3. Roll the mixture into bite-size balls and roll them lightly on the plate of dried coconut to coat. Transfer to the baking sheet and refrigerate for 1 hour before eating. Store leftovers in a sealed container in the refrigerator for 1 to 2 weeks.

Peanut Butter Chocolate Balls

Makes 10

¼ cup quick oats

¼ cup peanut butter

1 tablespoon hemp seeds

1 tablespoon ground
flaxseeds

1½ tablespoons raw cacao
powder

½ teaspoon vanilla extract

¼ cup pitted dates

½ teaspoon sea salt

1 tablespoon water

¼ cup mini chocolate chips

These easy-to-make balls are not only a nice dessert but also a great on-the-go snack idea. Just pack them in an airtight container and take them with you. Their fiber and protein make them a perfect midafternoon snack when you might be tempted to reach for something a little less healthy. Do your best to have no more than 2 balls in one sitting. After all, someone else may want some too. Perfect for any day other than your Low-Carb Days.

1. In a food processor, combine the oats, peanut butter, hemp seeds, flaxseeds, cacao, vanilla, dates, and sea salt. Process for 20 to 30 seconds. Add the water and process again until the mixture comes together. Stir in the chocolate chips.

2. Line a baking sheet with parchment paper. Roll the peanut butter mixture into bite-size balls, place them on the baking sheet, and refrigerate for 1 hour before eating. These can be stored in the refrigerator for 2 to 3 days.

Banana Oat Cookies

Makes 10

3 ripe bananas

1½ cups gluten-free rolled
   oats

¼ cup almond butter

½ tablespoon honey

2 tablespoons hemp seeds

1 tablespoon ground
   flaxseeds

1 teaspoon vanilla extract

½ teaspoon sea salt

1 teaspoon ground
   cinnamon

½ cup unsweetened
   shredded coconut

⅓ cup chopped walnuts or
   almonds

¼ cup dried fruit of your
   choice (optional)

These cookies are so easy to whip together. If you're ever feeling like a little treat (other than on your Low-Carb Days) and want something quick that you can make with what you probably already have in your pantry, these cookies fit the bill. Remember, the riper the bananas, the sweeter the taste. And if you're using extremely ripe bananas (borderline black), then I wouldn't even bother adding any honey or dried fruit.

1. Preheat the oven to 350°F. Line a baking sheet with parchment paper.

2. In a large bowl, mash the bananas with a fork. Stir in the oats, almond butter, honey, hemp seeds, flaxseeds, vanilla, salt, and cinnamon until well combined. Fold in the coconut, nuts, and dried fruit (if using). Let the mixture sit for 5 minutes to thicken.

3. Using a spoon, drop dollops of the mixture onto the baking sheet and flatten them with a fork. Bake for 20 to 25 minutes, or until golden brown. Cool on the baking sheet, then enjoy!

Salted Peanut Butter–Chocolate Pudding with Coconut Whipped Cream

Makes 3 to 4 servings

2 ripe bananas

½ cup cacao powder

1 tablespoon maple syrup

1 tablespoon ground
flaxseeds

3 tablespoons coconut oil,
melted

2 tablespoons creamy
peanut butter

1 teaspoon sea salt

1 can (14 ounces) full-fat
coconut milk, chilled

1 tablespoon ground
cinnamon

As you can probably tell by its name, this recipe should be reserved for your 1-Day Feast or the occasional Regular-Cal Day. It's pretty rich yet still based on real, whole-food ingredients. I feel odd saying this, but we peanut butter plus chocolate lovers should thank Harry Burnett Reese—the man who invented the Reese's Peanut Butter Cup in the 1920s. I'm not a supporter of Big Food conglomerates, but you have to tip your hat to the marriage of these two wonderful ingredients. Following each bite with a swig of almond milk comes pretty close to heaven for me. How about you?

1. In a food processor or blender, combine the bananas, cacao, maple syrup, flaxseeds, and coconut oil. Blend until smooth. Scoop into 3 or 4 small bowls. Top each bowl with a spoonful of peanut butter and a sprinkle of the salt.

2. Meanwhile, scoop the solid coconut cream at the top of the can of coconut milk into a large bowl. Discard the liquid. Add the cinnamon, then beat with an electric mixer for about 2 minutes, or until somewhat fluffy.

3. Add a scoop of coconut cream to each bowl and enjoy.

Caramelized Peaches
with Coconut Whipped Cream

Feast Approved

Makes 2 servings

2 large peaches, halved

2 tablespoons butter, melted

5 teaspoons ground cinnamon, divided

4 teaspoons honey

1 can (14 ounces) full-fat coconut milk

Peaches drenched in butter, honey, and cinnamon—sign me up! Don't be afraid of the butter. The French have been drowning their food in butter since the beginning of time, and their cuisine and physiques are to be envied. This is a richer dessert, so I would save it for your 1-Day Feast or Regular-Cal Day. Do your best to share. It will be hard, but you can do it.

1. Preheat the oven to 350°F. Line a baking sheet with parchment paper.

2. Place the peach halves on the baking sheet. Top each with ½ tablespoon of the butter, 1 teaspoon of the cinnamon, and 1 teaspoon of honey. Bake the peaches for 20 to 25 minutes, or until tender and golden brown around the edges. Remove from the oven and allow to cool slightly.

3. Meanwhile, scoop the solid coconut cream at the top of the can of coconut milk into a large bowl. Discard the liquid. Add the remaining 1 teaspoon cinnamon, then beat with an electric mixer for 2 minutes, or until somewhat fluffy.

4. Place a scoop of coconut cream on top of each peach half, and enjoy.

Flourless Orange–Almond Cake

Makes 10 servings

6 eggs, separated

½ cup coconut palm sugar

2 teaspoons grated orange peel

1 teaspoon vanilla extract

1 teaspoon ground cinnamon

2 cups ground almonds or almond flour

2 tablespoons freshly squeezed orange juice

1 tablespoon unsweetened shredded coconut

¼ cup slivered almonds

If you're in the mood for something a little lighter, then this delicious cake will be right up your alley. Almond flour is one of the best flours to use for baking because it's naturally very moist and not very heavy. The result is a lighter, fluffier texture. This cake is also a good dessert option for your Low-Carb Days and goes really well with a nice herbal tea.

1. Preheat the oven to 350°F. Grease a 9" round baking pan and line it with parchment paper.

2. In a large bowl, beat together the egg yolks, sugar, orange peel, vanilla, and cinnamon until thickened, about 5 minutes. Fold in the ground almonds or almond flour and orange juice.

3. In a separate bowl, beat the egg whites for 1 minute, or until soft peaks form. Stir half of the egg whites into the egg yolk mixture until combined, then fold in the remaining egg whites and combine. Scrape the batter into the baking pan.

4. Bake until the cake pulls away from the side of the pan, about 35 minutes. Run a knife around the edge and let cool on a rack for 10 minutes. Sprinkle the coconut and slivered almonds on top and serve.

Apple-Strawberry Crumble

Makes 4 servings

2 cups halved strawberries

1 apple, cored and cubed

2 tablespoons maple
syrup, divided

1 tablespoon vanilla
extract

2 teaspoons ground
cinnamon

1 cup gluten-free rolled
oats

½ cup unsweetened
shredded coconut

¼ cup coconut oil, melted

½ teaspoon sea salt

¼ cup butter, melted

1 can (14 ounces) coconut
milk

Did your grandma ever make you apple crumble when you were young? Can you still taste the memories? I don't have that memory, but my wife does, and I think many others do as well. With this healthier apple and strawberry version, you can enjoy this dessert—guilt-free—on a Feast Day or Regular-Cal Day. This is a big win for me since my kryptonite is strawberry-rhubarb pie, which, as you probably know, doesn't do a body good with all that lard, sugar, and who knows what else. So yes, I created this crumble recipe for my own guilty pleasure, but I think you'll enjoy it too.

1. Preheat the oven to 350°F. In a large bowl, stir together the strawberries, apple, 1 tablespoon of the maple syrup, vanilla, and cinnamon. Scrape the mixture into a greased 8" x 8" baking dish.

2. In a separate bowl, mix together the oats, coconut, oil, remaining 1 tablespoon maple syrup, and salt. Add the melted butter and combine well, then sprinkle over the strawberry-apple mixture.

3. Bake until the topping is golden brown and the filling is bubbly, about 30 minutes. Let stand a few minutes, then serve in bowls and pour the coconut milk over the top.

Strawberry Pudding

Makes 2 servings

2 cups hulled strawberries
+ additional chopped
strawberries for garnish
(optional)

½ cup blueberries

1 ripe avocado

1 teaspoon vanilla extract

¼ cup water

¼ cup cashews

4 drops liquid stevia

½ teaspoon sea salt

This rich and creamy pudding could even be used as a breakfast, if you like. It's loaded with great nutrition, and the avocado and cashews cut the sweetness of the berries. Whenever you decide to enjoy this, I would recommend topping it with Coconut Whipped Cream (page 130) simply because the combination is awesome. No other reason. Enjoy.

In a high-powered blender, combine the 2 cups strawberries, blueberries, avocado, vanilla, water, cashews, liquid stevia, and salt. Blend for 20 to 30 seconds, or until smooth. Serve in bowls. Garnish with additional chopped strawberries, if desired.

Coco-Chocolate Brownies

Feast Approved

Makes 12

¾ cup cocoa powder

1 cup pumpkin seed flour
(make by grinding raw
pumpkin seeds in a
coffee grinder)

½ cup unsweetened
shredded coconut

Pinch of sea salt

2 teaspoons arrowroot or
tapioca starch/tapioca
flour

½ cup applesauce

3 tablespoons coconut oil,
melted

1 tablespoon maple syrup
or honey

2 teaspoons vanilla extract

2 teaspoons water

Have you ever thought of using pumpkin seed flour for baking? If not, I think you'll really enjoy this dessert, especially if you're looking for an alternative to almond flour. Pumpkin seeds carry a lot of nutritional value, including a ton of zinc, and the taste of this flour is almost neutral, so it doesn't detract from the chocolaty goodness of the brownies. However, if you don't have pumpkin seeds on hand, you can use almond flour instead. For an added touch, top each brownie with Coconut Whipped Cream (page 130) and a sprig of mint.

1. Preheat the oven to 350°F. Lightly grease a 9" x 9" baking dish.

2. In a large bowl, mix together the cocoa, flour, coconut, salt, and arrowroot or tapioca.

3. In a separate bowl, mix together the applesauce, oil, maple syrup or honey, vanilla, and water. Pour into the flour mixture and stir everything together.

4. Pour the batter into the baking dish, pat it down with a spatula, and bake for 20 minutes, or until a toothpick inserted in the brownies comes out clean. Let cool on a wire rack, then cut into 12 squares.

Chocolate Chip Oatmeal Cookies

Feast Approved

Makes about 10

1½ cups almond flour

1 teaspoon baking soda

½ teaspoon kosher salt

¼ teaspoon ground
   cinnamon

1 cup semisweet
   chocolate chips

½ cup maple syrup

2 cups gluten-free
   old-fashioned oats

1 cup shredded coconut

4 tablespoons coconut oil,
   at room temperature

2 eggs, beaten

1 teaspoon vanilla extract

2 tablespoons ground
   flaxseeds

I remember the days when I would stay up late watching random TV shows while mindlessly drenching one chocolate chip cookie after another in a glass of milk, then allowing the softened goodness to sit in my mouth while I savored the moment. I'm not a very nostalgic person, but it's funny how memories of food can change that. Instead of eating store-bought cookies loaded with junk, fix these homemade ones that are so much better. And they take just a few minutes to prepare. I know you'll enjoy them too.

1. Preheat the oven to 375°F. Lightly brush a baking sheet with coconut oil.

2. In a large bowl, stir together the flour, baking soda, salt, cinnamon, chocolate chips, maple syrup, oats, coconut, oil, eggs, vanilla, and flaxseeds. Once well combined, use a large spoon to scoop the batter onto the baking sheet. Flatten, if desired, with your hand or the bottom of a glass.

3. Bake for 20 minutes. Cool on a rack, then enjoy.

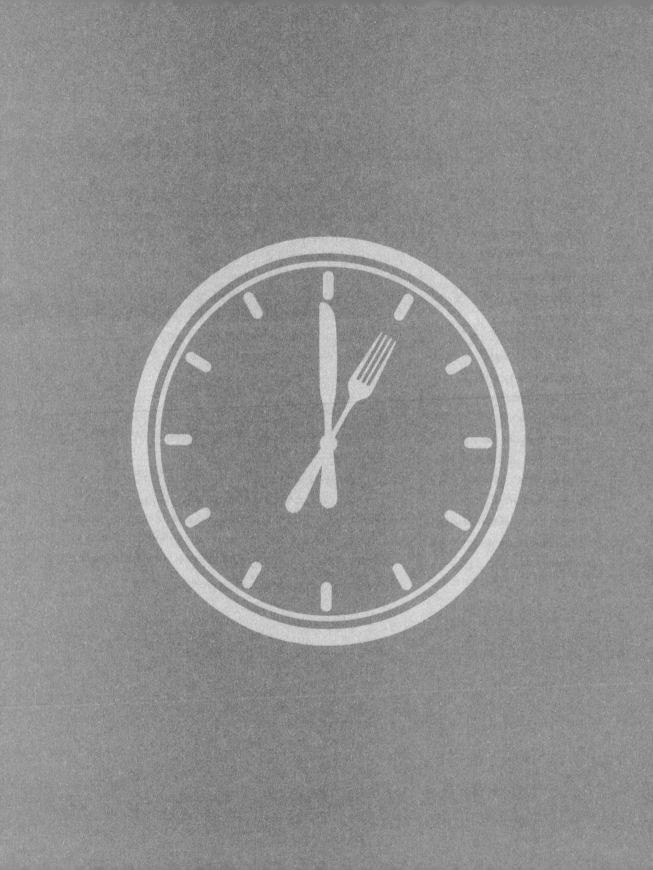

Chapter 13

The 10-Day Metabolic Reset

WANT ME TO HOLD YOUR HAND and help reset and turbocharge your metabolism so you can start burning away those extra pounds, all while enjoying gourmet-style meals? Then read on, and let's take this delicious 10-day journey together.

10 Days to a Leaner You

In *The All-Day Fat-Burning Diet,* I helped thousands of women and men lose up to 5 pounds per week in just 21 days. Some experienced more weight loss, others a little bit less. But everyone saw and felt noticeable improvements. With this 10-Day Metabolic Reset, I'm going to help you achieve similar results, but in half the time. Can you commit to just 10 days? I bet you can. And to be honest, you won't want to stop after you see and feel the difference.

What follows is a 10-day meal plan that incorporates many of the recipes in this cookbook, conveniently organized around the 5-Day Food-Cycling Formula. If you want a done-for-you, no-thinking-required plan to kick things off and help reset your metabolism, then follow this plan. Once you've eaten your way through these 10 days, you can either repeat the cycle, revert to the 21-day meal plan in the original All-Day Fat-Burning Diet, pick and choose your favorite recipes to enjoy within the 5-day food cycle, or simply eat whichever recipe you like whenever you want. After all, this is not a diet that you follow for just a few weeks, but rather a way of eating that you can live with forever.

As you go through these 10 days, if a particular recipe doesn't appeal to you, then simply find another one in this cookbook that does, so long as it's suitable for the appropriate day. For example, substitute another recipe designated "Low Carb" for one you don't like. Choosing a "Feast Approved" meal on a Low-Carb Day would defeat the magic of our 5-Day Food-Cycling Formula.

One final note on meal frequency: Here, I've laid out your meals based on a three-meal-per-day schedule. However, you don't *have* to eat three meals. You can have two, four, or whatever else will best suit your needs and schedule. If you do decide to eat more or fewer meals, just remember to choose recipes for the appropriate day (to choose recipes designated "Low Carb" for your Low-Carb Days, for example).

Also, as I've mentioned before, breakfast isn't always necessary. Plus breakfast doesn't have to be eaten when you first get out of bed. Breakfast is simply the first meal of your day—whatever time that may be. For me, that often ends up being around noon, since I spend many mornings in a fasted state. So listen to your body to know when you're truly hungry. If you'd like a downloadable grocery list for the 10-Day Metabolic Reset (along with some more cool stuff), just go to www.alldayfatburningdiet.com/cookbook/stuff.

Larissa Goes from Yo-Yo Dieting to Losing 10 Pounds of Excess Baby Weight and 6 Inches

"Since my early teens, I have almost always been on one diet or another. I would lose weight, then gain it all back. I was the epitome of a yo-yo dieter! Over the past several years (after getting married and having two babies close together), I gave up diets and focused more on healthy eating. My weight stabilized, but I still needed to lose about 15 pounds. I always hit the same plateau on the scale no matter what I did! Besides the extra pounds, I've also been plagued for years with frequent headaches, dizzy spells, and back pain from tight muscles. I was already thinking about going gluten-free when I saw someone on Facebook recommend the *All-Day Fat-Burning Diet*. I thought, why not?

"I am so glad I decided to purchase this book! It has changed my life! Yuri thoroughly explains the science behind the nutrition in a way that is easy to understand. I also appreciate how he understands that each body is different and advocates for ultimately listening to your body. In the first 3 weeks, I lost over 10 pounds (finally breaking through that plateau!) and over 6 total inches from my waist, lower abs, hips, and thighs. But even more wonderful is the fact that my headaches, dizzy spells, and back pain have diminished. (I don't even have any cramps or low-back aching during my periods!) My energy has also increased, which is a big deal, since I am a full-time stay-at-home mom to my toddlers.

"And did I mention that the recipes are delicious? Even the picky eaters in my family have fallen in love with a few of them. This is not 'just another diet' but rather a lifestyle that I have gratefully adopted and will continue to live by for the sake of my health."

Day 1: Low-Carb Day

Breakfast—Whipped Coconut Cream and Berries (page 86)

Lunch—Kale and Avocado Teaser Caesar Salad (page 143)

Dinner—Bacon-Tomato Zucchini Pasta (page 185)

Day 2: 1-Day Feast

Breakfast—Fried Egg Breakfast Hash (page 89)

Lunch—Rainbow Rice Bowl (page 157)

Dinner—Chicken and Apricot Tagine with Saffron Quinoa
(page 189)

Day 3: 1-Day Fast

N/A

Day 4: Regular-Cal Day

Breakfast—Protein-Packed Morning Muesli with Applesauce (page 91)

Lunch—Plant-Powered Protein Soup (page 170)

Dinner—Green Chickpea Tahini Bowl (page 159)

Day 5: Low-Cal Day

Breakfast—Spinach-Pear Smoothie (page 100)

Lunch—Vermicelli Garden Bowl (page 156)

Dinner—Tasty Thai Stir-Fry (page 197)

Day 6: Low-Carb Day

Breakfast—Hemp Seed Porridge (page 90)

Lunch—Kaleslaw (page 144)

Dinner—Pan-Seared Salmon with Sugar Snap Peas and Avocado
Salad (page 188)

Day 7: 1-Day Feast

Breakfast—Homemade Chocolate Granola (page 95)

Lunch—Lentilicious Salad (page 145)

Dinner—Italian Sausage and Roasted Root Vegetables (page 205)

Day 8: 1-Day Fast

N/A

Day 9: Regular-Cal Day

Breakfast—Prosciutto-Wrapped Asparagus with Fried Eggs (page 93)

Lunch—Apple-Kale Salad with Poppy Seed Dressing (page 138)

Dinner—Steak Frites (page 193)

Day 10: Low-Cal Day

Breakfast—Citrus Refresher (page 110)

Lunch—No-Cook Ginger Thai Soup (page 177)

Dinner—Chicken and Vegetable Curry (page 196)

Kris Reverses Her Anemia and Gets Off Her Thyroid Meds

"I began this diet with the goal of getting as healthy as possible before a major back surgery. I've been disabled for a decade and unable to work out much, so while I did not have a lot of weight to lose, my BMI was not good at all. I was also being treated for anemia and thyroid dysfunction. After my fourth week on the program, my presurgery blood work came back, and my anemia was gone. I was also able to stop my thyroid meds! My measurements are shrinking, and my weight is going down! By following Yuri's instructions, taking the toxic load off my body and following this simple program, my BMI is back to where it was 25 years ago, in college. Yuri's research and work is genius, and I can't thank him enough!"

I'm on a Mission . . . Want to Join Me?

The year is 2040, and our A-team of motivated game changers has helped create a world where 100 million people now have the knowledge and means to live a healthier and more fulfilling life. They are financially secure (or free) and fueled by good nutrition and daily movement. Each person has a deep understanding of his or her body and has access to the technology and resources to be his or her own "doctor" instead of relying on drugs or the broken medical system.

This is just part of the vision I have for our future. And I've been put on this planet to help make that a reality. But I can't do it alone. I need motivated, health-conscious people like you to help us spread the word and be part of this mission to empower and free more people from a life of frustration, scarcity, confusion, and lack of access to important health resources.

The best thing you can do to help reach our goal is to simply let your light shine. Be your true self and commit to becoming better each and every day. In doing so, you will become an inspiration to those around you. In time, they'll be motivated to make positive changes for themselves too. That's how true, lasting change occurs. To begin this journey together, join our community and get simple and clear guidance on how to live your healthiest life at YuriElkaim.com.

Let's do this together!

In Conclusion

My goal has always been and will continue to be to empower you to take control of your health and your future. I hope you're excited about these recipes and, more importantly, the fundamental understanding you will gain by making them, which will allow you to create your own masterpieces in the kitchen.

Yes, it's great to have done-for-you recipes and meal plans. But it's even more powerful if you experience and understand how various foods and ingredients work together, which flavor combinations work in different situations, and how to eat in a way that resonates with your body. There is no one-size-fits-all diet.

You are unique. That means you need to constantly experiment and discover what works best for you. And be okay with the fact that your desires and needs may change over the course of your life.

Wherever you are now, I look forward to hearing about your success, and my hope is that you become an inspiration in the kitchen to yourself and those around you. Remember, knowing how to prepare your own food—that is simple, healthy, and delicious—is one of the most fundamental life skills we must develop for lasting health and leanness.

Your friend and coach,

Yuri

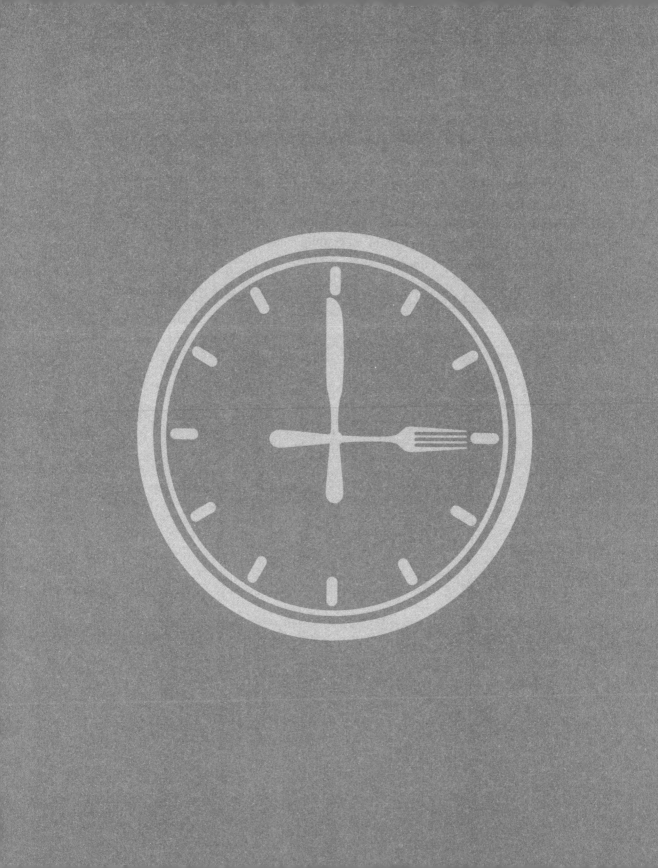

Endnotes

Introduction

1 http://journals.cambridge.org/action/displayAbstract;jsessionid=C46B7F6E31746BE61D4ACD17604BDE73.journals?aid=8621878&fileId=S136898001200136X

Chapter 1

1 Katmarzyk, P., et al. (2009). Sitting Time and Mortality from All Causes, Cardiovascular Disease, and Cancer. *Medicine & Science in Sports & Exercise* 41(5): 998–1005.

2 Rash, J., et al. (2011). Gratitude and Well-Being: Who Benefits the Most from a Gratitude Intervention? *Applied Psychology: Health and Well-Being* 3(3), 350–69.

Chapter 2

1 Duhigg, C. (2014). *The Power of Habit: Why We Do What We Do in Life and Business.* New York: Random House Trade Paperbacks.

2 Judah, G., et al. (2012). Forming a Flossing Habit: An Exploratory Study of the Psychological Determinants of Habit Formation. *British Journal of Health Psychology* 18(2): 338–53.

3 Fogg, BJ. www.foggmethod.com/.

4 Lally, P., et al. (2009). How Are Habits Formed: Modelling Habit Formation in the Real World. *European Journal of Social Psychology* 40(6): 998–1009.

5 Baumeister, Roy F., Ellen Bratslavsky, Mark Muraven, and Dianne M. Tice. (1998). Ego Depletion: Is the Active Self a Limited Resource? *Journal of Personality and Social Psychology* 74(5): 1252–65.

6 Ibid.

7 Danziger, S., et al. (2011). Extraneous Factors in Judicial Decisions. *Proceedings of the National Academy of Sciences* 108(17): 6889–92.

8 Gaillot, M., and R. Baumeister. (2007). The Physiology of Willpower: Linking Blood Glucose to Self-Control. *Personality and Social Psychology Review* 11(4): 303–27.

Chapter 3

1 Rosenblat, G. (2011). Polyhydroxylated Fatty Alcohols Derived from Avocado Suppress Inflammatory Response and Provide Non-Sunscreen Protection against UV-Induced Damage in Skin Cells. *Archives of Dermatological Research* 303(4): 239–46.

2 Opalinski, Heather A. (2012). High Fructose Corn Syrup, Mercury, and Autism—Is There a Link? *Journal of the American Academy of Special Education Professionals.* (Spring–Summer 2012): 122–38.

3 Takigawa, T., and Y. Endo. (March 2006) The Effects of Glutaraldehyde Exposure on Human Health. *Journal of Occupational Health* 48(2): 75–87.

4 Behall, K., et al. (2005). Consumption of Both Resistant Starch and β-Glucan Improves Postprandial Plasma Glucose and Insulin in Women. *Diabetes Care* 29(5): 976–81.

5 Robertson, D., et al (2005). Insulin-Sensitizing Effects of Dietary Resistant Starch and Effects on Skeletal Muscle and Adipose Tissue Metabolism. *American Journal of Clinical Nutrition* 82(3): 559–67.

6 Keenan, M., et al. (2006). Resistant Starch Reduces Abdominal Fat More than Energy Dilution with Nonfermentable Fiber. *FASEB Journal* 20 (Meeting Abstract Supplement).

7 Jenkins, D., et al. (2011). The Relation of Low Glycaemic Index Fruit Consumption to Glycaemic Control and Risk Factors for Coronary Heart Disease in Type 2 Diabetes. *Diabetologia* 54(2): 271–79.

8 Joseph, J. A., et al. (1999). Reversals of Age-Related Declines in Neuronal Signal Transduction, Cognitive, and Motor Behavioral Deficits with Blueberry, Spinach, or Strawberry Dietary Supplementation. *Journal of Neuroscience* 19(18): 8114–21.

9 Youdim, K. A., et al. (2000). Polyphenolics Enhance Red Blood Cell Resistance to Oxidative Stress: In Vitro and in Vivo. *Biochimica et Biophysica Acta* 1523: 117–22.

10 Lau, F. C., D. F. Bielinski, and J. A. Joseph. (2007). Inhibitory Effects of Blueberry Extract on the Production of Inflammatory Mediators in Lipopolysaccharide-Activated BV2 Microglia. *Journal of Neuroscience Research* 85: 1010–17.

11 Afshin, A. (July 1, 2014). Consumption of Nuts and Legumes and Risk of Incident Ischemic Heart Disease, Stroke, and Diabetes: A Systematic Review and Meta-Analysis. *American Journal of Clinical Nutrition* 100(1): 278–88.

12 Salehi-Abargouei, A., et al. (2015). Effects of Non-Soy Legume Consumption on C-Reactive Protein: A Systematic Review and Meta-Analysis. *Nutrition* 31(5): 631–39.

13 Hermsdorff, H. (2011). A Legume-Based Hypocaloric Diet Reduces Proinflammatory Status and Improves Metabolic Features in Overweight/Obese Subjects. *European Journal of Nutrition* 50(1): 61–69.

14 Hung, H. C., et al. (2004). Fruit and Vegetable Intake and Risk of Major Chronic Disease. *Journal of the National Cancer Institute* 96(21): 1577–84.

15 Traka, M., and R. Mithen. (2008). Glucosinolates, Isothiocyanates and Human Health. *Phytochemistry Reviews* 8(1): 269–82.

16 Cohen, J. H., A. R. Kristal, and J. L. Stanford. (2000). Fruit and Vegetable Intakes and Prostate Cancer Risk. *Journal of the National Cancer Institute* 92: 61–68.

17 Larsson, S. C., N. Hakansson, I. Naslund, et al. (2006). Fruit and Vegetable Consumption in Relation to Pancreatic Cancer Risk: A Prospective Study. *Cancer Epidemiology, Biomarkers & Prevention* 15: 301–5.

18 Zhang, C. X., S. C. Ho, Y. M. Chen, et al. (2009). Greater Vegetable and Fruit Intake Is Associated with a Lower Risk of Breast Cancer among Chinese Women. *International Journal of Cancer* 125: 181–88.

19 Khandouzi, N., et al. (2015). The Effects of Ginger on Fasting Blood Sugar, Hemoglobin A1c, Apolipoprotein B, Apolipoprotein A-I and Malondialdehyde in Type 2 Diabetic Patients. *Iranian Journal of Pharmaceutical Research* 14(1): 131–40.

20 Black, C., et al. (2010). Ginger (Zingiber officinale) Reduces Muscle Pain Caused by Eccentric Exercise. *Journal of Pain* 11(9): 894–903.

21 Dulloo, A. G. (March 1996) Twenty-Four-Hour Energy Expenditure and Urinary Catecholamines of Humans

Consuming Low-to-Moderate Amounts of Medium-Chain Triglycerides: A Dose-Response Study in a Human Respiratory Chamber. *European Journal of Clinical Nutrition* 50(3): 152–58.

22 White, M., et al. (1999). Enhanced Postprandial Energy Expenditure with Medium-Chain Fatty Acid Feeding Is Attenuated after 14 Days in Premenopausal Women. *American Journal of Clinical Nutrition* 69(5): 883–89.

23 Kaunitz, H. (1971). Dietary Use of MCT in "Bilanzierte Ernaehrung in der Therapie," K. Lang, W. Fekl, and G. Berg, eds. George Thieme Verlag, Stuttgart.

24 Baba, N., E. F. Bracco, J. Seylar, and S. A. Hashim. (1981). Enhanced Thermogenesis and Diminished Deposition of Fat in Response to Overfeeding with Diets Containing Medium Chain Triglycerides. *American Journal of Clinical Nutrition* 34: 624.

25 Johansson, K., et al. (January 2014). Effects of Anti-Obesity Drugs, Diet, and Exercise on Weight-Loss Maintenance after a Very-Low-Calorie Diet or Low-Calorie Diet: A Systematic Review and Meta-Analysis of Randomized Controlled Trials. *American Journal of Clinical Nutrition.* 99(1): 14–23.

26 Leidy, H. Acute Satiety Effects of Sausage/Egg-Based Convenience Breakfast Meals in Premenopausal Women. Presented at Obesity Society's Annual Scientific Meeting, November 14, 2013, Atlanta.

Chapter 5

1 Higgins, J. (2004). Resistant Starch: Metabolic Effects and Potential Health Benefits. *Journal of AOAC International* 87(3): 761–68(8).

Chapter 11

1 Bes-Rastrollo, M. (2006). Olive Oil Consumption and Weight Change: The SUN Prospective Cohort Study. *Lipids* 41(3): 249–56.

2 Razquin, C., et al. (2009). A 3 Years Follow-Up of a Mediterranean Diet Rich in Virgin Olive Oil Is Associated with High Plasma Antioxidant Capacity and Reduced Body Weight Gain. *European Journal of Clinical Nutrition* 63: 1387–93.

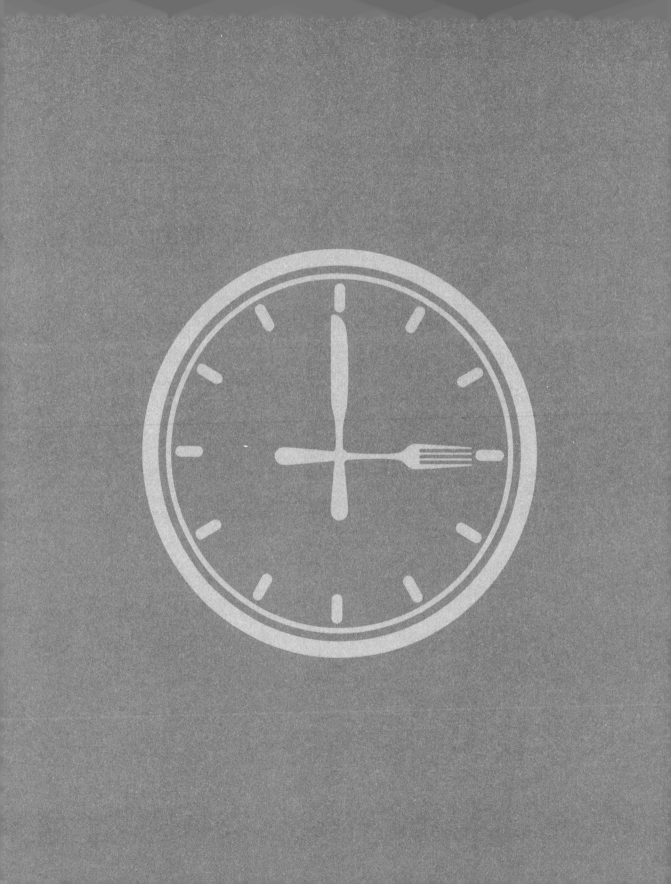

Index

Underscored page references indicate boxed text. An asterisk (*) indicates recipe photos are shown in the color inserts.

Chicken
Broccoli-Chicken Skillet,* 202
Chicken and Apricot Tagine with Saffron Quinoa,* 189
Chicken and Vegetable Curry, 196
Fast and Flavorful Chicken and Veggies, 190
Finger Lickin' Chicken Salad, 194
Honey-Sesame Chicken Stir-Fry, 204
Zucchini Pesto Pasta with Sliced Chicken, 186
Chickpeas
benefits of, 64–65
Chickpeas in Coconut Milk, 123
Curried Chickpea Salad,* 152
Flavorful Moroccan Chickpea Soup,* 173
Green Chickpea Tahini Bowl, 159
Hummus, 128
Spicy Garlic Oven-Roasted Chickpeas, 153
Chocolate
Chocolate Chip Oatmeal Cookies,* 219
Chocolate Protein Smoothie, 106
Coco-Chocolate Brownies,* 218
Homemade Chocolate Granola,* 95
Peanut Butter Chocolate Balls, 211
Salted Peanut Butter–Chocolate Pudding with Coconut Whipped Cream,* 213
Chopped ingredients, 48
Cinnamon
Apple-Cinnamon Chia Seed Pudding, 88
metabolism boost from, 73

Circadian rhythms, 5, 58–60
Coconut
Coco-Chocolate Brownies,* 218
Coconut milk
Apple-Strawberry Crumble,* 216
Banana Oat Cookies, 212
Caramelized Peaches with Coconut Whipped Cream,* 214
Cherry-Coconut Granola, 94
Coco-Goji Balls, 210
Coconut-Mango Chia Seed Pudding, 87
Coconut Whipped Cream, 130
Crazy Coconut Smoothie, 109
fat in, 17
Salted Peanut Butter–Chocolate Pudding with Coconut Whipped Cream,* 213
Tasty Thai Stir-Fry, 197
Whipped Coconut Cream and Berries,* 86
Coconut oil
fats in, 51–52, 53
metabolism boost from, 74, 76, 76
virgin, cold-pressed, 81
Coffee, 15, 15
Collard greens
Raw Collard Wrap recipes, 164–65
Competency, four stages of, 32–33
Cookware, 46–47
Corn oil, 51–52, 53
Cortisol, 3, 5, 15, 57, 58
Coumarin, 73
CPR Method, 31, 33–37
Cravings, 9, 11, 23, 27, 31, 77
Cruciferous vegetables, metabolism boost from, 74

Cucumbers
Lemon-Oregano Shrimp with Tomato, Cucumber, and Olive Salad,* 192
Cue, in habit formation, 33–36, 35
Curcumin, 74
Currants
Quinoa, Kale, and Current Salad, 141
Curry, 196
Cutting board, 48–49

D

Dessert recipes, 209–19
Detoxification, 69, 74
Diabetes, 14, 16
A1C decrease with ginger, 72
carbohydrates and, 61, 62, 63, 66
Diced ingredients, 48
Digestive enzymes, 10
Dips, snacks, and toppings recipes, 127–35
Discipline, 41–42
Disinfectants, 57
Dopamine, 34
Dressing for kale salads, 75
Dutch oven, 46

E

Eating
bingeing, 57
frugally, 7
meal number per day, 15–16
Eating habits, 31–43
creating tiny habits, 36
how habits are formed, 32–33
making habits stick, 37–38
myth about habits, 39–42